BREAST PATHOLOGY
Benign Proliferations, Atypias & In Situ Carcinomas

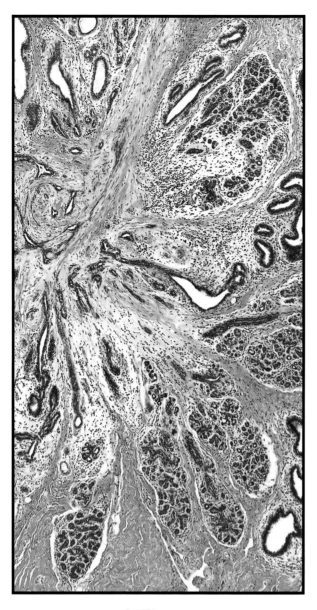

BREAST PATHOLOGY
Benign Proliferations, Atypias & In Situ Carcinomas

Robert E. Fechner, MD
Professor of Pathology
University of Virginia Health Sciences Center
Charlottesville, Virginia

Stacey E. Mills, MD
Professor of Pathology
University of Virginia Health Sciences Center
Charlottesville, Virginia

ASCP Press
American Society of Clinical Pathologists · Chicago

Cover and Title Page
Figure 7-5. Radial scar with prominent central collagen.
Ductules entrapped in the scar are distorted.

Library of Congress Cataloging in Publication Data

Fechner, Robert E.
    Breast pathology: benign proliferations, atypias, and in situ
carcinomas / Robert E. Fechner, Stacey E. Mills.
    Includes bibliographical references.
    Includes index.
    ISBN 0-89189-298-2
    1. Breast—Tumors—Diagnosis. 2. Breast—Biopsy, Needle.
3. Breast—Histopathology. I. Mills, Stacey E. II. Title.
    [DNLM: 1. Breast—pathology. 2. Breast Neoplasms—pathology.
3. Carcinoma in Situ—pathology. 4. Fibrocystic Disease of Breast—
pathology. 5. Hyperplasia—pathology. WP 815 F291b]
RC280.B8F43 1990
616.99′44907583—dc20
DNLM/DLC
for Library of Congress   90-647
                                                              CIP

Printed in Hong Kong by Everbest Printing Co Ltd.

94 93 92 91 90   5 4 3 2 1

CONTENTS

PREFACE

This monograph is intended to discuss and generously illustrate part of the enormous morphologic spectrum that benign, atypical, and in situ neoplastic breast tissue can assume. The focus of the text is a patient-oriented, risk assessment philosophy. We believe that this approach emphasizes the proper role of the "1990s" surgical pathologist in the care of patients undergoing breast biopsy and appropriately de-emphasizes the bipolar "Is it benign or is it malignant?" approach. The reading lists at the end of each chapter are as up to date as the time limits of publication would allow, but are not meant to be an exhaustive bibliography. Rather, they should serve to guide the reader to sources that discuss aspects of our text in greater detail.

It is our goal to provide a large number of illustrations, representing the diverse range of problematic entries to a greater degree than is typical of other single sources. Many ducts and lobules illustrated herein are first shown at scanning power, as they would be encountered during the perusal of a microscopic slide, followed by higher magnification, as if one were "dropping down" for a closer look. Although this approach requires a large number of figures, we believe that it best approximates the manner in which such lesions are encountered during our day-to-day practice.

We are indebted to Nancy J. Kriigel, whose expert secretarial and editorial skills greatly aided in the preparation of this monograph. In addition, we wish to thank Joshua Weikersheimer, Director, and Stephen Borysewicz, Editor, ASCP Press, for their patience, encouragement, and helpful suggestions.

Robert E. Fechner, MD
Stacey E. Mills, MD

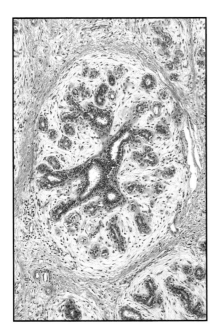

Philosophy of Risk Assessment

During the past decade, there have been dramatic improvements in radiographic techniques for imaging and localizing small, often nonpalpable abnormalities of the breast. The resultant, growing number of mammographically directed biopsy specimens has placed increasing demands on pathologists to properly diagnose a variety of noninvasive epithelial abnormalities. The major purpose of this book is to extensively illustrate these changes. The alterations fall into two major groups. First are those benign conditions that are of little clinical significance except for their tendency to be confused with in situ or invasive carcinoma.

The second group includes the spectrum of noninvasive epithelial proliferations ranging from "typical" hyperplasias to in situ lobular or ductal carcinomas. These proliferations are associated with variable risks for the development of invasive carcinoma. The concept of risk assessment is a major improvement in the pathologist's approach to noninvasive breast disease. This approach recognizes that women with histologically distinctive ductal and lobular proliferations can be assigned a risk for the subsequent development of invasive carcinoma as compared with an age-matched general population. Information permitting such an assessment is generated by large, retrospective and prospective studies of women receiving no additional therapy after biopsy. The studies by

Page and associates provide the largest number of patients with the most objective and applicable criteria for dividing noninvasive breast changes into clinically relevant degrees of risk. Excluding carcinoma in situ, these authors divided the microscopic findings of fibrocystic changes into categories of *nonproliferative, proliferative without atypia,* and *proliferative with atypia.* Women without proliferative changes have not been shown to be at statistically increased risk of developing invasive carcinoma, as compared with an age-matched general population. Women with proliferative disease without atypia are at approximately twice the risk, and lesions diagnosed as atypical hyperplasia place women at five times the risk of developing invasive disease. The risks associated with ductal and lobular carcinoma in situ are addressed in other studies, and each type carries approximately a tenfold increase in the frequency of invasive carcinoma if the patient receives no additional therapy.

Clinicians can combine these pathologic risk factors with a variety of clinical factors including patient age, family history of breast carcinoma, and pregnancy and lactational status. The resultant overall assessment can then provide a rational basis for discussing management options with the patient.

It should be borne in mind that the cited data regarding the risks of invasive carcinoma are far from the final word on this topic, and many important questions remain to be addressed. For example, much of these data are derived from premammographic studies in which the presence of a palpable mass led to a biopsy. Does lobular carcinoma in situ incidentally found in a palpable mass carry the same risk of invasive carcinoma as lobular carcinoma in situ discovered by a mammographically directed biopsy of a nonpalpable abnormality? Breast tissue was often sparsely sampled in older studies. Does atypical intraductal hyperplasia detected in one of three slides from an incompletely sectioned 4-cm biopsy specimen carry the same risk for invasive carcinoma as atypical intraductal hyperplasia detected in one of 20 slides from a completely sectioned, mammogram-generated biopsy specimen of the same size? Even in the premammographic era, complete sectioning of a breast biopsy specimen was shown to double the yield of carcinoma in situ, when compared with the conventional, less than total sampling of the same specimen (Patchefsky et al).

A number of studies suggest that carcinoma in situ is a highly prevalent lesion in the clinically benign breast tissue of adult women. One study of reduction mammoplasty specimens found lobular carcinoma in situ in six (8%) of 70 women over the age of 40 years (Bondeson et al). Two to 40 tissue blocks were submitted. Autopsy studies of the breasts of women who did not have detectable breast cancer during life have yielded similar results. Kramer and Rush made an average of 40 slides per breast from women over the age of 70 years. Four (5.7%) of 70 had intraductal carcinoma. Nielsen et al (1984) took 57 to 166 blocks from the breasts of 77 women without previous clinical breast cancer. Fourteen cases (18%) had ductal carcinoma in situ, lobular carcinoma in situ, or both. Another study by Nielsen et al (1987) found that 18% of women less than 55 years old had ductal or lobular carcinoma in situ. Using the subgross radiographic method of breast examination, Alpers and Wellings found that nine (10%) of 91 women over the age of 20 years had ductal carcinoma in situ in autopsy specimens. This included two of the 32 women between 20 and 39 years old.

These data also raise many currently unanswerable questions. How many of the foci would have been detected by mammography during life? How long had the lesions been present? In the autopsy studies, did the lesions in older women arise late in life and thereby not have sufficient time to evolve into an invasive cancer?

Recent studies strongly suggest that not only the quality but the quantity of ductal and lobular proliferations must be evaluated before arriving at a risk factor for subsequent invasive carcinoma following biopsy alone. If these trends continue, then data derived from older studies of large, palpable lesions may have limited applicability. If such is the case, we may be overestimating the clinical importance of qualitatively identical, smaller lesions being found with increasing frequency by mammographically directed biopsies.

Although the above considerations challenge the available data on the *absolute risk* of invasive carcinoma based solely on qualitative changes, the risk assessment approach, as discussed below, remains a valid one, provided that we think in terms of *relative risk*. This approach has several effects on practicing pathologists. In large part, it eliminates the binary clinicopathologic decision of: "If it's cancer the patient needs a major procedure, if it isn't cancer, all is well." The histologic continuum of noninvasive breast proliferations does not always allow "all or none" distinctions. For the pathologist, this more realistic view appropriately de-emphasizes formerly heavily weighted diagnostic distinctions, such as the difference between atypical lobular hyperplasia ("Sounds benign, no problem!") and lobular carcinoma in situ ("Carcinoma! The patient needs a mastectomy!"). We now realize, of course, that both lesions carry an increased risk for invasive carcinoma, although the majority of patients in both groups will never develop life-threatening disease.

Because there are no abrupt morphologic changes in the continuum of lobular and ductal proliferations, and because we lack markers to identify fully transformed (malignant) cells in situ, the diagnosis of borderline atypical epithelial proliferations must remain a matter of opinion. Accordingly, different pathologists will vary in their interpretation of such images. These differences do not constitute "mistakes," providing the pathologists place the lesion in closely related categories. For example, if one pathologist views a borderline lesion as atypical hyperplasia and another interprets it as ductal carcinoma in situ, this should not cause undue concern. The patient may be viewed as having a relative risk of invasive cancer that is at least as great as for atypical hyperplasia and may be as great as for carcinoma in situ. A serious diagnostic problem exists only when opinions differ greatly, as when one pathologist considers a lesion to be carcinoma in situ and another considers it to represent hyperplasia without atypia. One of the two pathologists in this situation has seriously overestimated or underestimated the risk of later invasive carcinoma.

To minimize errors of the latter type, we have provided prototypical examples of various epithelial proliferations to serve as "benchmarks" for comparison with problematic cases. For risk evaluations derived from prior studies to be meaningful, diagnostic criteria must be applied as uniformly as possible, given the limitations imposed by a disease continuum. For example, "atypical hyperplasia" must be reserved for the approximately 4% of breast biopsy specimens in the premammographic era containing marked cytologic or architectural abnormalities that approached but fell short of carcinoma in situ. This percentage may increase in mammographically directed biopsies, as noted recently by Urbanski et al. The term "atypical hyperplasia" should not be applied to "funny-looking" proliferations that lack any of the specific cytologic abnormalities characteristic of carcinoma in situ.

Risk assessment also requires the segregation of microscopically distinctive proliferations. It is no longer satisfactory to lump a host of proliferations under the rubric of "fibrocystic disease." The published conclusions from a recent consensus meeting state that the various microscopic components of "fibrocystic disease" must be specified if an accurate evaluation of the risk for invasive carcinoma is to be obtained (Hutter, 1986).

REFERENCES

Alpers CE, Wellings SR. The prevalence of carcinoma in situ in normal and cancer-associated breasts. Hum Pathol 1985;16:796-807.

Bartow SA, Pathak DR, Black WC, et al. Prevalence of benign, atypical, and malignant breast lesions in populations at different risk for breast cancer. A forensic autopsy study. Cancer 1987;60:2751-2760.

Bondeson L, Linell F, Ringberg A. Breast reductions. What to do with all of the tissue specimens? Histopathology 1985;9:281-285.

DuPont WD, Page DL. Risk factors for breast cancer in women with proliferative breast disease. N Engl J Med 1985;312:146-151.

Dupont WD, Page DL. Relative risk of breast cancer varies with time since diagnosis of atypical hyperplasia. Hum Pathol 1989;20:723-725.

Hutter RVP. Goodbye to 'fibrocystic disease.' N Engl J Med 1985;312:179 (editorial).

Hutter RVP. Consensus statement. Is 'fibrocystic disease' of the breast precancerous? Arch Pathol 1986;110:171-173.

Kramer WM, Rush BF Jr. Mammary duct proliferation in the elderly. A histopathologic study. Cancer 1973;31:130-137.

Nielsen M, Jensen J, Andersen J. Precancerous and cancerous breast lesions during lifetime and at autopsy. A study of 83 women. Cancer 1984;54:612-615.

Nielsen M, Thomsen JL, Primdahl S, et al. Breast cancer and atypia among young and middle-aged women. A study of 110 medicolegal autopsies. Br J Cancer 1987;56:814-819.

Page DL. Cancer risk assessment in benign breast biopsies. Hum Pathol 1986;17:871-874.

Page DL, DuPont WD, Rogers LW, Rados MS. Atypical hyperplastic lesions of the female breast. A long-term follow-up study. Cancer 1985;55:2698-2708.

Page DL, VanderZwaag R, Rogers LW, et al. Relation between component parts of fibrocystic disease complex and breast cancer. JNCI 1978;61:1055-1063.

Patchefsky AS, Potok J, Hoch WS, Libshitz HI. Increased detection of occult breast carcinoma after more thorough histologic examination of breast biopsies. Am J Clin Pathol 1973;60:799-804.

Urbanski S, Jensen HM, Cooke G, et al. The association of histological and radiological indicators of breast cancer risk. Br J Cancer 1988;58:474-479.

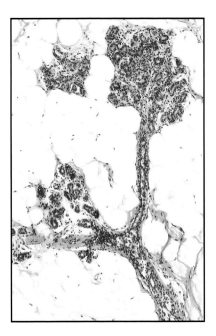

NORMAL ANATOMY, VARIATIONS, AND IATROGENIC CHANGES

The epithelial portion of the adult breast consists of lobules and the ducts that connect them to the nipple. Different terms have been applied to the several components of this system. In this book, we utilize the terminology of Wellings et al (1975) to describe the microscopic anatomy of the breast. The lobule consists of ductules that are the smallest, blindly ending, epithelial-lined structures of the breast (Figures 2-1, 2-2). Each ductule opens into a slightly larger channel called the *terminal duct*. A terminal duct therefore has an intralobular segment that is in continuity with each of the ductules, and then the terminal duct exits the lobule as a single channel (Figure 2-3). Rarely, terminal ducts enter directly into a large duct (Figure 2-4). More commonly, the extralobular portion of the terminal duct ends when it merges with another terminal duct to form a small subsegmental duct (Figures 2-5, 2-6). The subsegmental ducts merge with one another, forming progressively larger ducts. The final 15 to 20 largest ducts of the breast that are located in the breast parenchyma immediately beneath the nipple and open onto its surface are called segmental, collecting, or *lactiferous* ducts. The collecting duct may expand just beneath the nipple to form an intramammary lactiferous sinus.

The collecting duct is the termination of a segment or lobe of the breast with its numerous lobules and smaller ducts. The segments presumably overlap or intertwine with one another, and they are not recognizable either at the time of surgery or on pathologic examination.

In the nonlactating breast, all of the lobules and ducts are lined by a single inner layer of epithelial cells and an outer layer of myoepithelium. The epithelial cells have round or ovoid nuclei and moderate to scant cytoplasm. The myoepithelial layer often appears discontinuous at the light microscopic level, when the nuclei are widely separated, and the cytoplasm is attenuated to the point of being indiscernible. When the myoepithelial cells are more prominent, they often have a zone of perinuclear clearing.

There is considerable variation in the appearance of different lobules, even on the same microscopic slide. One lobule may be populated by plump epithelial and myoepithelial cells, whereas the adjacent lobule may have cells with small nuclei, virtually no cytoplasm, and narrow lumina. Most lobules are sectioned so that only the ductules are seen. Occasionally, a fortuitous section will disclose the terminal duct. Usually the lobule has a loose fibrous stroma that surrounds and separates the individual ductules and forms a narrow cuff at its periphery. Lobules may, however, lack this loose perilobular connective tissue and directly abut adipocytes. There also may be adipocytes within the lobule.

Menstrual Cycle Changes

Much of the histologic variation in the mammary lobules of premenopausal women may be due to hormonally mediated changes that correlate with the menstrual cycle. As a general statement, during the proliferative phase of the cycle the lobules tend to be small, mitoses are uncommon, and the intralobular stroma is condensed. In the secretory phase, the lobules and their ductules increase in size with a loose and edematous intralobular stroma. During this phase, the epithelium contains mitotic figures and vacuolated cytoplasm. During the perimenstrual portion of the cycle, there may be sloughing of ductular epithelium, accompanied by a lymphocytic infiltrate. The lobule then reverts to its appearance in the proliferative phase. There are inconsistencies in different studies regarding these cyclic changes. From a practical standpoint, however, cyclic changes do not create diagnostic problems.

Pregnancy and Lactation

The changes that occur in pregnancy and lactation represent the ultimate functional activity of the breast. During pregnancy, there is an enormous proliferation and enlargement of lobules. By the third trimester, the epithelium accumulates fat droplets, and the luminal portion of the cytoplasm is often vacuolated. The intralobular stroma appears to be diminished as the proliferating lobules closely approximate one another.

During lactation the epithelial cells are vacuolated and have small cytoplasmic blebs on their luminal borders. The cytoplasm is generally less abundant than during pregnancy because of the apocrine-type secretion of milk. After luminal cytoplasm has been shed with secretions, the remaining nuclei protrude into the lumen of the ductule, resulting in a "hobnailed" appearance. It takes at least 3 months after cessation of lactation for the breast to return to its nonlactational histologic appearance.

Postmenopausal Breast

The lobules of the breast gradually atrophy after menopause in most women. The epithelial and myoepithelial cells become smaller, and the ductular lumina may be imperceptible. The loose intralobular connective tissue seen in the premenopausal breast becomes progressively collagenized and less cellular. It is likely that some lobules completely disappear. The persistence of atrophic lobules may reflect the longevity of some ductular cells or, possibly, continuing replacement of cells in some lobules.

The combination of postmenopausal atrophy and dense collagenization may isolate small cellular clusters or individual epithelial cells. This change, combined with the loss of normal lobular architecture, can lead to confusion with carcinoma. The small, bland nature of the epithelial nuclei, together with a lack of elastosis or an active desmoplastic reaction, should permit distinction. Although most breasts undergo atrophic changes after menopause, many do not. The entire spectrum of premenopausal lobular appearances can be seen in postmenopausal women, including elderly women beyond the age of 75 years. Wellings et al (1976) consider the persistence of mature mammary lobules after menopause to be an abnormality associated with an increased risk for subsequent development of carcinoma.

CLEAR CELL AND PREGNANCY-LIKE CHANGE

Clear Cell Change

Barwick et al described cytoplasmic clearing in the cells lining mammary ducts and lobules. Affected women ranged in age from 35 to 82 years. There was no discernible pattern regarding parity, lactation, or hormonal therapy. Many examples were incidental findings in breasts removed because of carcinoma, but there was no clear-cut association with cancer.

Clear cell change involves either epithelium or myoepithelium. The epithelial cells are often enlarged to three to four times their normal size (Figures 2-7, 2-8). The cytoplasm is finely granular or grainy, with occasional coarse, irregularly distributed, eosinophilic granules. There may be completely clear vacuoles of varying size. The ductal or ductular lumina are typically maintained, and may contain eosinophilic granules similar to those seen within the cytoplasm. Some epithelial nuclei in clear cell change are small, dense, and pyknotic-appearing, whereas others are of normal size with fine, uniform chromatin.

Ultrastructurally, granules of varying size are present. Some are membrane-delimited with an internal, electron-dense beading. Others are dense and amorphous. These granules are similar in appearance to those studied in the breasts of pregnant or lactating rodents. In the animal models, the granules have been shown to contain protein and lipid. The lipid is presumably removed during tissue processing and accounts for the clear cell change.

Clear cell change can also involve myoepithelial cells (Figure 2-9). Cytoplasmic and nuclear changes are similar to those seen in epithelial cells, with the exception that the altered myoepithelial cells lack cytoplasmic granularity. Myoepithelial cells may be affected without involvement of the overlying epithelium. It may be difficult in some instances to determine whether clear cell change is involving myoepithelium, epithelium, or both (Figure 2-10).

Clear cell change differs from pregnancy-like change in that most nuclei in the former condition are small, and the hobnailed, secretory appearance of pregnancy-like change is absent. Moreover, although there may be some dilatation of ductules involved by clear cell change, it is typically less than is seen in pregnancy-like change.

Pregnancy-Like Change

Occasionally, breast lobules may contain dilated ductules with epithelial changes identical to those seen in pregnancy or lactation (Figures 2-11, 2-12). By definition, this pregnancy-like change occurs in women who are neither pregnant nor lactating. Some women are nulliparous. The frequency of pregnancy-like change is remarkably constant in both autopsy and surgical series. Frantz et al and Sandison described it in 3.1% and 3.7%, respectively, of women at autopsy. Kiaer and Andersen noted the change in 3% of consecutive surgical specimens removed for either benign or malignant breast disease. There appears to be no association with carcinoma or any specific form of benign breast disease. Occasionally, patients have been taking antihypertensive, antipsychotic, or estrogenic medications (Tavassoli and Yeh).

Pregnancy-like change usually affects only part or all of a single lobule or, at most, a few adjacent lobules. The remainder of the breast typically lacks this alteration. The cells of pregnancy-like change can form small "micropapillary" tufts that protrude into lumina containing amorphous secretory material. The cytoplasm is vacuolated and may be abundant or form only a narrow rim around the nucleus. Nuclei have smudged, densely hyperchromatic chromatin and range from two to seven times the diameter of normal epithelial cells. Often, nuclei are located at the apical end of the cell, imparting a hobnailed appearance (Figure 2-12).

The enlarged cells with hyperchromatic nuclei and, in some instances, an increased nuclear to cytoplasmic ratio, may suggest intraductal carcinoma. This suspicion is heightened if there is secretory material within the ducts intermixed with exfoliated nuclei and thereby resembling comedocarcinoma. The hobnailed appearance of the individual cells, the vacuolization of the cytoplasm regardless of its quantity, and the lack of well-developed comedo-type necrosis should allow distinction. So-called hypersecretory ductal carcinoma in situ (see page 109) also resembles pregnancy-like change because of the tufting of cells and their protrusion into lumina. Hypersecretory carcinoma, however, involves large ducts and not the slightly dilated lobules affected by pregnancy-like change.

IATROGENIC CHANGES

Radiation therapy is finding increasing use in the treatment of in situ and invasive carcinoma of the breast. Women who have received radiation therapy must be evaluated for local recurrence of the original carcinoma, as well as the development of a new neoplasm. New abnormalities detected by palpation or mammography usually lead to biopsy of the irradiated breast. The various effects of radiation can complicate the interpretation of these biopsy specimens.

Radiation most strikingly alters previously normal stroma and epithelium. Radiation changes in the extralobular stroma include irregular zones of dense collagen containing enlarged, atypical fibroblasts, as are seen in radiation-induced injury of any organ. The intralobular stroma appears to be especially sensitive to radiation. It becomes sparsely cellular or totally acellular and assumes a densely collagenized or hyalinized appearance (Figure 2-13). There may be fat necrosis with its typical components of lipophages, giant cells, lymphocytes, and plasma cells. This reaction may be so extensive as to clinically mimic recurrent carcinoma (Clarke et al).

Prominent vascular alterations, identical to those that occur in other irradiated tissues, may be seen in the breast. Myointimal proliferation in small, muscular arteries may narrow or completely obliterate the lumen. Myxoid degeneration of the intima, degeneration of the smooth muscle of the media, and adventitial fibrosis also occur. Capillaries may be lined by enlarged endothelial cells that bulge into the lumina.

The terminal duct–lobular unit appears to contain the epithelial cells that are most sensitive to radiation change. Lobules may become atrophic, with a few residual cells lacking lumen formation as the only remnants of ductules. Myoepithelial cells appear to be more radioresistant, and may be prominent compared with the atrophic epithelium. The atrophic lobules are usually the ones with the most conspicuous stromal fibrosis, as described above. Other lobules may have intact, larger than normal cells, due to nucleomegaly, accompanied by variable increases in the quantity of cytoplasm (Figures 2-14 to 2-17). The nuclei in these altered cells are hyperchromatic and may have small nucleoli. The cytoplasm is eosinophilic and has a ground-glass appearance or is delicately vacuolated. The epithelial changes may be focal, involving only a portion of one or more ductules. Sometimes, the enlarged epithelial cells protrude into the lumen, and because of their size, may partly or completely obliterate it. The lining cells of the terminal duct may be unaltered, minimally involved, or totally affected.

Extralobular ducts can have all of the cytologic alterations described above, but they tend to be involved far less commonly. As with the lobules, only a portion of a duct may be abnormal. The cells maintain their polarity and are cohesive without necrosis. Ductal changes are most often seen in patients who also have extensive alterations in the terminal duct–lobular unit.

The differential diagnosis of radiation atypia includes lobular and ductal carcinoma in situ. The cytologic features of radiation-damaged nonneoplastic cells may overlap with those of lobular carcinoma in situ. In this situation, features such as the degree of cellular proliferation must be utilized. Radiation change may result in narrowed or obliterated ductular lumina, but it does not produce distention of the involved ductule by increased numbers of epithelial cells. The altered cells in terminal or larger ducts lie in their normal location without tufting or other evidence of proliferation, thus excluding a diagnosis of ductal carcinoma in situ. Radiation-altered cells occasionally may be seen in foci of ductal

or lobular hyperplasia, raising the question of atypical hyperplasia. In such instances, similar-appearing radiation-altered cells should be sought in nonproliferative areas to aid in this distinction.

The susceptibility of individual breasts to radiation damage is highly variable. Schnitt et al found that radiation changes could not be correlated with the presence or absence of carcinoma elsewhere in the specimen, the age of the patient, the radiation dose, or the time between radiation therapy and the subsequent biopsy. Some patients had received adjuvant chemotherapy, and this could not be discerned as having an additive or special effect.

The effect of radiation on the cytologic features of preexistent carcinoma has not been extensively studied. Most of the data available are from patients who have had mastectomies after failure of radiation treatment. As a general statement, the carcinoma appears identical before and after irradiation. This applies to both infiltrating and intraductal carcinomas. Occasionally, an irradiated tumor has cells with multiple nuclei, or there may be necrosis that was not seen in the pretreatment biopsy specimen. Such differences could be due, however, to the limited sampling of the original, unirradiated specimen.

Fully diagnostic ductal and lobular carcinoma in situ can, of course, be found in the breasts of women who have received radiation therapy for carcinoma (Figure 2-18). In our experience, the diagnostic criteria that are applied to an unirradiated breast biopsy specimen also can be applied to in situ abnormalities in the irradiated breast. We have seen both ductal and lobular carcinoma in situ accompanied by other ducts or lobules having the radiation changes described above. The distinction between radiation changes and in situ neoplasia has been clear-cut in these instances.

Fine Needle Aspiration Tracts

Many carcinomas of the breast are diagnosed by fine needle aspiration. Sections of the subsequently excised tumor often include the needle tract. Depending on the interval between aspiration and excision, a spectrum of changes may be present. Tissue removed within a few days of aspiration shows the needle tract to be a freshly hemorrhagic zone containing neutrophils, fat necrosis, and small amounts of hemosiderin. As the interval increases, the tract becomes filled with proliferating fibroblasts, greater quantities of hemosiderin, and diminished numbers of inflammatory cells.

We have seen one case in which a needle tract was identified in the mastectomy specimen from a patient with comedocarcinoma. Clumps of intact, extraductal tumor cells cytologically identical to the comedocarcinoma were intermixed with neutrophils and foamy histiocytes. There was no desmoplastic response and the neoplastic cells were "floating" within the inflammatory reaction (Figures 2-19, 2-20). These features led us to conclude that the cells had been artifactually dislodged from the ducts by the aspiration needle, and that they did not represent invasive carcinoma.

Cautery Effect

Electrocautery instruments similar to those used for bladder or prostate surgery are being applied more frequently in the biopsy of breast tissue. This may result in considerable distortion of cytologic detail in breast specimens, just as it does in genitourinary tract material. The thermal artifact may render the epithelium of ducts or lobules cytologically uninterpretable (Figures 2-21, 2-22). Most damage occurs within 1 mm of the surface of the specimen, and, particularly in cases of ductal carcinoma in situ, this can make it difficult to distinguish margin involvement.

In addition to the cautery-induced cytologic artifacts, there may be architectural distortion. Thus, areas of normally complex sclerosing adenosis may appear even more disorganized, mimicking infiltrating carcinoma. The loss of cytologic detail in such histologically deranged foci may prevent a rational interpretation, and the pathologist must be careful to avoid overdiagnosis or underdiagnosis. Fortunately, cautery artifact does not deeply penetrate the tissue and, in most instances, does not interfere with microscopic evaluation.

Epithelial Telescoping

The physical disruption and compression of ductal epithelium during surgical manipulation may result in an appearance evocative of papillary carcinoma or hyperplasia. Close inspection, however, will show that such foci consist of layers of cytologically normal epithelium. The compressed and folded or "telescoped" epithelium may form discontinuous strands within the duct lumen or the strands may buckle into the lumen while maintaining their continuity with the original duct wall (Figures 2-23, 2-24).

REFERENCES

Anderson TJ, Ferguson DJP, Raab GM. Cell turnover in the 'resting' human breast. The influence of parity, contraceptive pill, age and laterality. *Br J. Cancer* 1982;46:376-382.

Barwick KW, Kashgarian M, Rosen PP. 'Clear-cell' change within duct and lobular epithelium of the human breast. *Pathol Annu* 1982;17(part 1):319-328.

Clarke D, Curtis JL, Martinez A, et al. Fat necrosis of the breast simulating recurrent carcinoma after primary radiotherapy in the management of early stage breast cancer. *Cancer* 1983;52:442-445.

Ferguson DJP. Intraepithelial lymphocytes and macrophages in the normal breast. *Virchows Arch A* 1985;407:369-378.

Ferguson DJP. An ultrastructural study of mitosis and cytokinesis in normal 'resting' human breast. *Cell Tissue Res* 1988;252:581-587.

Ferguson DJP. Ultrastructural characteristics of the proliferative (stem?) cells within the parenchyma of the normal 'resting' breast. *Virchows Arch A* 1985;407:379-385.

Ferguson DJP, Anderson TJ. Morphological evaluation of cell turnover in relation to the menstrual cycle in the 'resting' human breast. *Br J Cancer* 1981;44:177-181.

Frantz VK, Pickren JW, Melcher GW, Auchincloss H Jr. Incidence of chronic cystic disease in so-called 'normal breasts.' A study based on 225 postmortem examinations. *Cancer* 1951; 4:762-783.

Frierson HF Jr, Fechner RE, Tabbarah S. Diagnostic pitfalls in the tissue reaction to fine needle aspiration. *Am J Clin Pathol* 1989;92: 534 (Abstract).

Humphrey LJ, Swerdlow M. Histologic changes in clinically normal breasts at postmortem examination. *Arch Surg* 1966;92:192-193.

Kiaer HW, Andersen JA. Focal pregnancy-like changes in the breast. *Acta Pathol Microbiol Scand A* 1977;85:931-941.

Longacre TA, Bartow SA. A correlative morphologic study of human breast and endometrium in the menstrual cycle. *Am J Surg Pathol* 1986;10:382-393.

Meyer JS. Cell proliferation in normal human breast ducts, fibroadenomas, and other ductal hyperplasias measured by nuclear labeling with tritiated thymidine. Effects of menstrual phase, age, and oral contraceptive hormones. *Hum Pathol* 1977;8:67-81.

Mills SE, Fechner RE. Focal pregnancy-like change of the breast. *Diagnost Gynecol Obstet* 1980;2:67-70.

Mills SE, Fraire AE. Pregnancy-like change of the breast. An ultrastructural study. *Diagnost Gynecol Obstet* 1981;3:187-191.

Rosen PP: Letter to editor (electrocautery effect). *Ann Surg* 1986;204:612-613.

Sandison AT. An autopsy study of the adult human breast. *Natl Cancer Inst Monogr* 1962;8:58-59.

Schnitt SJ, Connolly JL, Harris JR, Cohen RB. Radiation-induced changes in the breast. *Hum Pathol* 1984;15:545-550.

Stirling JW, Chandler JA. The fine structure of the normal, resting terminal ductal-lobular unit of the female breast. *Virchows Arch A* 1976;372:205-226.

Tavassoli FA, Yeh IT. Lactational and clear cell changes of the breast in nonlactating, nonpregnant women. *Am J Clin Pathol* 1987;87:23-29.

Vina M, Wells CA: Clear cell metaplasia of the breast. A lesion showing eccrine differentiation. *Histopathology* 1989;15:85-92.

Vogel PM, Georgiade NG, Fetter BF, et al. The correlation of histologic changes in the human breast with the menstrual cycle. *Am J Pathol* 1981;104:23-34.

Wellings SR, Jensen HM, DeVault MR. Persistent and atypical lobules in the human breast may be precancerous. *Experientia* 1976;32:1463-1465.

Wellings SR, Jensen HM, Marcum RG. An atlas of subgross pathology of the human breast with special reference to possible precancerous lesions. *JNCI* 1975;55:231-273.

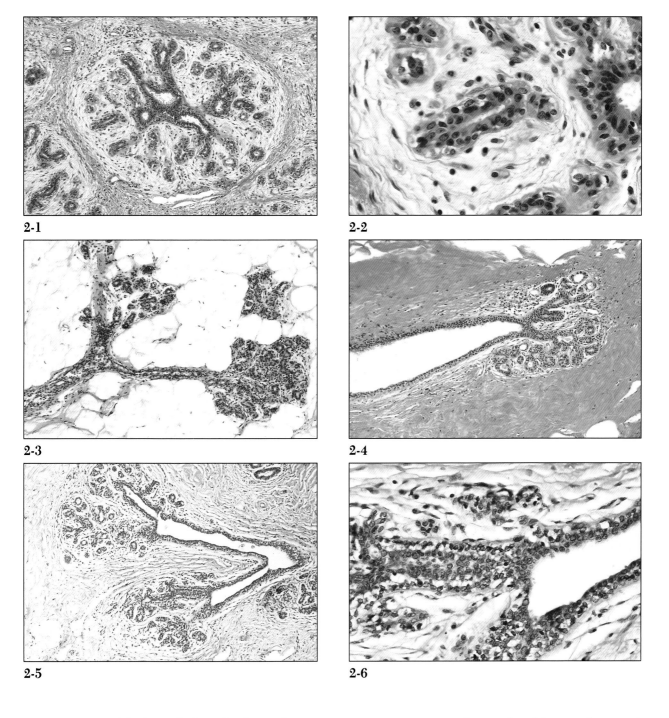

2-1

2-2

2-3

2-4

2-5

2-6

Figure 2-1. A lobule with ductules located peripherally around the intralobular segment of the terminal duct. Intralobular stroma is often looser than its extralobular counterpart.

Figure 2-3. The extralobular segment of terminal ducts from two lobules join at the lower left portion of the field. As can be seen, terminal ducts vary considerably in length.

Figure 2-5. Four lobules and their associated terminal ducts are sectioned in varying planes. Two subsegmental ducts from these terminal ducts fuse at the right of the field. This forms a larger branch of the subsegmental duct system.

Figure 2-2. Ductules are lined by two layers of cells. The outer, myoepithelial layer may be indistinct and often appears discontinuous.

Figure 2-4. Rarely, terminal ducts enter directly into a large duct.

Figure 2-6. Higher magnification of Figure 2-5 shows tangential sectioning of terminal ducts. This common phenomenon must not be mistaken for hyperplasia.

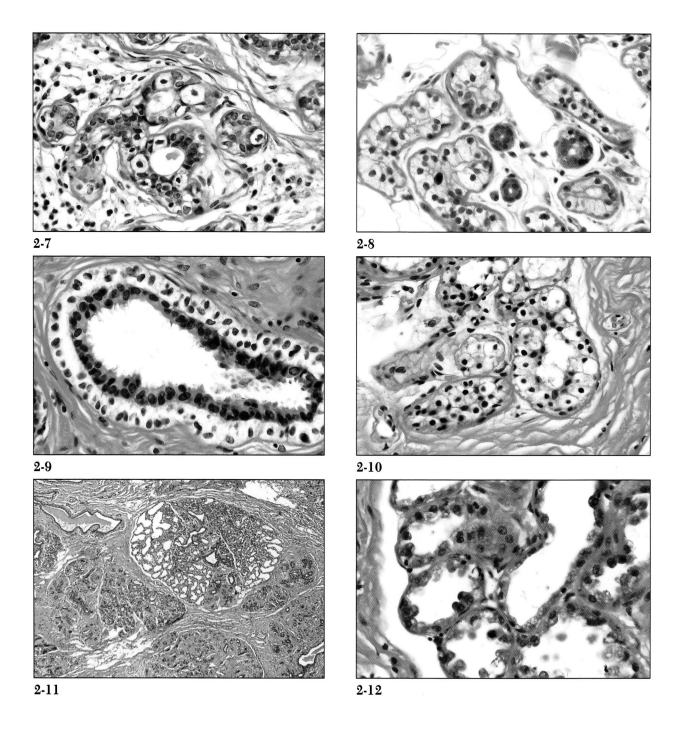

2-7

2-8

2-9

2-10

2-11

2-12

Figure 2-7. Clear cell change may involve isolated cells of the ductule. Note that the nuclei of the clear cells are slightly smaller and denser than normal. The nuclear and cytoplasmic features differ from those of lobular carcinoma in situ (pages 156 and 157).

Figure 2-9. Clear cell change is conspicuous in the myoepithelial cell layer.

Figure 2-11. Cluster of lobules in the upper portion of the field demonstrates the focal, dilated lumina characteristic of pregnancy-like change.

Figure 2-8. More extensive involvement of ductules by clear cell change can be contrasted with the residual normal ductules located centrally. The clear and nonclear epithelial cells have almost identical nuclear features.

Figure 2-10. Often it is difficult to determine if clear cell change involves epithelium, myoepithelium, or both.

Figure 2-12. The cells of pregnancy-like change have vacuolated cytoplasm. The nuclei are often at the luminal edge of the cell, creating a "hobnail" appearance.

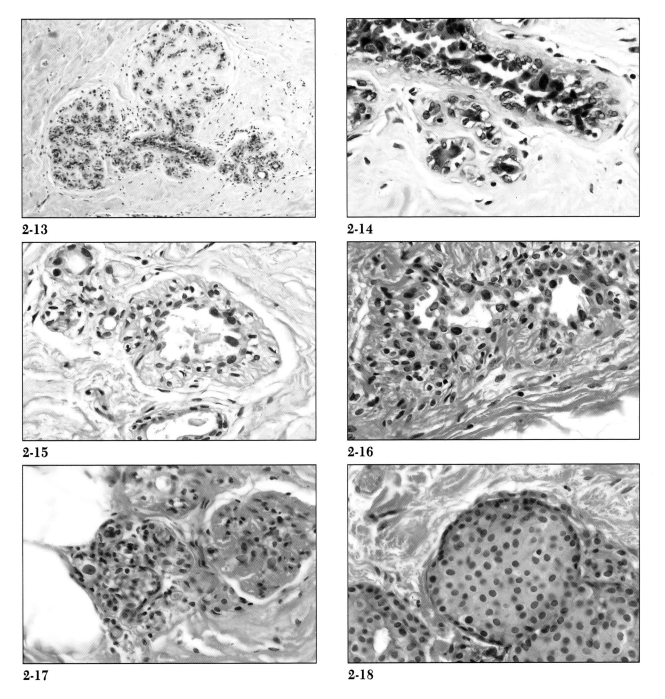

2-13

2-14

2-15

2-16

2-17

2-18

Figure 2-13. Tissue excised from patient who had received high-dose radiation therapy for invasive carcinoma 8 months earlier. The lobules are sparsely cellular and have hyalinized intralobular stroma.

Figure 2-15. Irradiated epithelial cells show focal, marked nucleomegaly with an increased nuclear-to-cytoplasmic ratio. Intraluminal cytoplasmic debris, as seen here, is occasionally present.

Figure 2-17. Sclerotic, irradiated ductule at the right contrasts with a more cellular ductule having isolated nucleomegaly at left.

Figure 2-14. The remnants of ductules contain an inner layer of epithelial cells with marked nuclear variation. The outer, myoepithelial cell layer is essentially normal.

Figure 2-16. Sometimes irradiated epithelial cells have variable but abundant eosinophilic cytoplasm. Note the prominent nuclear variation.

Figure 2-18. The same irradiated breast seen in Figure 2-17 also contained lobular carcinoma in situ. The diagnostic features of lobular carcinoma in situ are retained, and can be contrasted with the previously illustrated radiation changes.

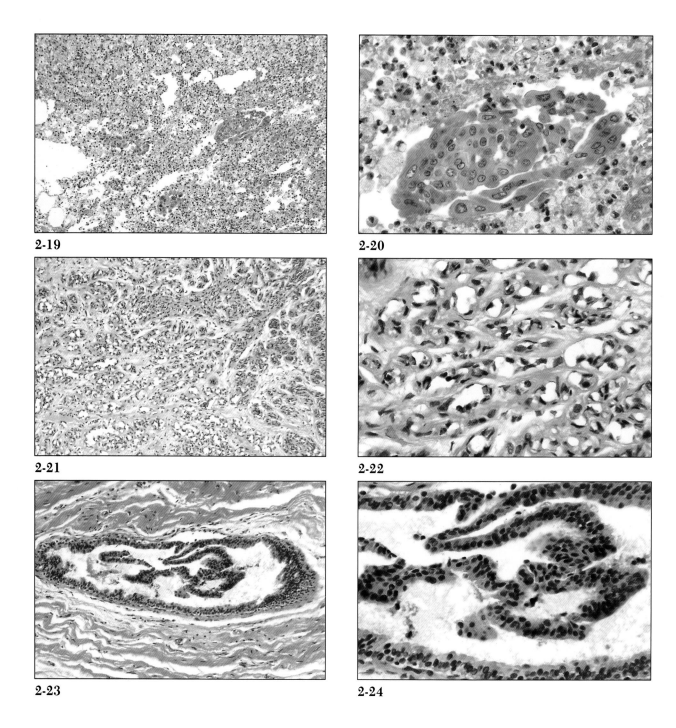

2-19

2-20

2-21

2-22

2-23

2-24

Figure 2-19. This patient with comedocarcinoma underwent fine needle aspiration. The subsequent mastectomy specimen had needle tracts containing free-floating neoplastic cells within a prominent inflammatory reaction.

Figure 2-21. Cautery-induced thermal artifact in sclerosing adenosis compounds the potentially difficult distinction from invasive carcinoma.

Figure 2-23. Mechanical disruption of ductal epithelium during biopsy may result in irregular strands of epithelial cells within the lumen. This may mimic hyperplasia at low power.

Figure 2-20. The tumor cells in the needle tract were cytologically identical to those in the comedocarcinoma. There is no desmoplastic response as would be seen with invasion. We believe that this represents needle-induced displacement of intraductal tumor and not invasive carcinoma.

Figure 2-22. Thermal artifact creates shrunken, densely hyperchromatic, and irregularly shaped nuclei. The cytoplasm is also frequently condensed around the nuclei.

Figure 2-24. At higher magnification, the disrupted epithelium is contiguous with and cytologically identical to the normal ductal lining.

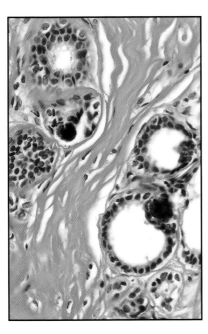

3

EVALUATION OF BIOPSY SPECIMENS, INCLUDING CALCIFICATIONS

Biopsy specimens from the breast have a spectrum of gross appearances that typically correlate with the clinical setting. For example, a 1- to 2-cm mass that is grossly obvious infiltrating carcinoma will usually be from a woman with a clinically palpable mass thought by the surgeon to be carcinoma. A biopsy specimen composed of firm fibrous tissue lacking gross evidence of carcinoma is likely to represent the "dominant lump" in a woman with diffuse fibrocystic changes. Such patients often have mammographic and physical findings that arouse suspicion of infiltrating carcinoma. On the other hand, the specimen that consists mainly of fat interspersed with soft fibrous tissue is almost always from a woman with no palpable mass and a mammographic abnormality either in the form of calcifications or a shadow.

Role of Frozen Section

The diverse sizes and appearances of breast specimens require considerable judgment in their management. One must never forget that the first priority is to arrive at the correct diagnosis. This priority is most often compromised by the inappropriate use of the frozen section. Frozen sectioning should never be done on breast tissue that is not grossly suggestive of invasive carcinoma or comedo-

carcinoma. We also recommend that small lesions (0.8 cm or less in greatest dimension) not be frozen, even if they are suggestive of invasive carcinoma. A small mass suggestive of cancer may be a radial scar, an adenosis tumor, or a ductal adenoma. Distinctions between these entities and carcinoma can be difficult or impossible on frozen section. Subsequent paraffin-embedded permanent sections of the frozen tissue may contain major freezing and crush artifacts that affect both architectural and cytologic details. These defects can render the permanent section not only suboptimal, but, occasionally, totally unsuitable for obtaining a definitive diagnosis, thus heedless or automatic use of frozen sectioning on a wide variety of breast specimens can render an extreme disservice to the patient.

Gross Lesion Suggestive of Carcinoma

A piece of tissue may be taken for frozen section from a specimen that appears grossly to be invasive carcinoma or comedocarcinoma with the proviso that adequate tissue must be available for unfrozen permanent sections and for receptor analysis. The purpose of a frozen section is to confirm the presence of carci-

16

noma or to suggest other diagnostic possibilities such as radial scar or sclerosing adenosis. In the latter situation, one does not want to submit tissue for receptor studies, because it may be necessary to examine the entire lesion to exclude carcinoma.

Approach to Specimens With Mammographic Calcifications Only

Tissue removed because of mammographically detected calcifications must be studied radiographically to confirm that the calcified area has been removed. This requires that the biopsy specimen remain intact to compare the specimen radiograph with the preoperative mammogram. Once the presence of the mammographically detected calcification has been verified, the pathologist must be certain that the calcified area is placed in one or more blocks that are specifically identified as containing the calcifications. Finally, calcium must be seen on the slides cut from these blocks, and this may require multiple sections. If the multiple sections fail to disclose calcium, the paraffin blocks can be x-rayed to see if the calcium is present deeper in the block. If it is still within the block, deeper levels are cut. Alternatively, the "missing calcifications" may represent calcium oxalate crystals not visible on routinely stained sections. Examination with polarized light will detect such crystals. They can also be stained with alizarin red S stain at pH 7.0 (Tornos et al).

Most of the calcifications seen on mammograms are readily identified on H&E-stained sections as dark blue calcium carbonate or calcium phosphate spherules. The smallest deposits of calcium may be intimately associated with either normal, hyperplastic, or neoplastic ductal or lobular epithelium. Many foci of lobular or ductal carcinoma in situ are devoid of calcium on microscopic sections, but nearby normal lobules or ducts contain calcium. Occasionally, the calcium lies free in the stroma near ducts or lobules. These may represent foci in which pre-existent epithelium became atrophic and disappeared.

There is general agreement that tissue blocks containing calcifications must be sampled until the calcium is identified microscopically, but the optimal approach to the remaining calcium-free tissue is unclear. This may be a large volume of tissue that, from a practical standpoint, cannot be completely sectioned. A study by Owings et al (1989) has indicated that almost all diagnostically important abnormalities are in the calcified area. Specifically, 35 of 36 carcinomas and eight of ten atypical hyperplasias were in the calcified foci. Thus, only one lesion of critical importance (a ductal carcinoma in situ) was in the tissue outside the calcified area, and could have been missed by less than total sectioning.

It is self-evident that when more sections are taken a microscopic abnormality is more likely to be found. In 1973, Patchefsky et al sectioned tissue from 244 breast biopsies, of which 149 specimens were able to be completely embedded in ten blocks or fewer. Three of these 149 cases had lobular or ductal carcinoma in situ. There were 95 cases that were originally sampled with ten blocks each, but had additional tissue that was not examined. The initial ten blocks from this group of 95 cases did not show carcinoma in situ, but when all of the remaining tissue was submitted, three (4%) of these 95 cases contained in situ carcinoma. Thus, in the entire group of 244 cases, the yield of lobular or ductal carcinoma in situ was doubled from 1.2% to 2.4% by embedding and sectioning all of the tissue. It is difficult to relate these data to current mammographic techniques and specimen examination. Two of the ductal carcinomas in situ that were found in the subsequently embedded tissue had calcium within them. It is possible that current mammographic techniques would have directed attention to these foci. Nevertheless, this study provides an approximation of the frequency with which additional sections identify important lesions.

For biopsies of mammographically detected calcifications, the cost-to-benefit ratio of completely sectioning only the calcified areas vs sectioning the entire, sometimes large specimen must be taken into account. Perhaps a reasonable approach to the calcium-free component is to apply the guidelines outlined below for biopsy specimens that completely lack calcification.

Approach to Grossly Benign Specimens Lacking Calcifications

The utility of specimen radiography for evaluating a "shadow" without mammographic calcifications is unclear. The arrangement of the "shadow" is almost always altered once it is excised and direct correlation with the mammogram may be difficult or impossible.

Furthermore, the number of sections to be taken from a biopsy specimen without a grossly invasive carcinoma is debatable. Obviously, the more sections that are taken, the greater the chance that noninvasive carcinoma will be found. Nonetheless, it is often not feasible to completely process a large biopsy specimen.

Schnitt and Wang have analyzed the likelihood that atypical hyperplasia or carcinoma in situ will be found in a breast biopsy specimen consisting only of grossly benign-appearing fibrofatty tissue. They have concluded that the detection of these abnormalities in fat is extremely uncommon. The only case in which a single focus of atypical lobular hyperplasia was found in fat was in a biopsy specimen that consisted exclusively of fat—a very rare occurrence. All of the other lesions were found in the fibrous component. They provided data suggesting that a maximum of ten blocks of fibrous parenchyma was a satisfactory approach to screening a specimen for atypical hyperplasia or carcinoma in situ. The likelihood that atypical hyperplasia or carcinoma in situ was present was related to specimen size. This is best explained by the fact that submitting more tissue from large specimens increases the chance of finding a lesion, as documented by Patchefsky et al. However, Schnitt and Wang noted that despite the high yield in large biopsy specimens, the number of blocks required to initially detect the lesion was small, and lesions appeared in one of the first ten blocks examined.

Their conclusions, based on careful mathematical analysis, are as follows. Submitting the fat is unnecessary. If the fibrous parenchymal component of a specimen can be encompassed in ten blocks or fewer, the entire specimen should be submitted. For larger specimens, ten blocks from the fibrous area can be submitted. If atypical hyperplasia or carcinoma in situ is identified, additional tissue can be submitted to see if there are other associated lesions, as well as to evaluate the margin of the excision (see below). If the specimen consists only of fat, ten blocks, or the entire specimen if encompassed in fewer blocks, is considered adequate.

Evaluation of Margins

The question of whether margins are involved with carcinoma (either invasive or noninvasive) has become relevant with the increasing use of radiation therapy as an alternative to mastectomy. Positive margins may affect whether the subsequent therapy will be radiation alone or wider local excision with or without radiation. As it is often unknown at the time of biopsy what form the subsequent therapy will take, all biopsies should be managed in a consistent manner.

Whether or not calcifications are present radiographically, the first step in the pathologic examination of a biopsy specimen is to coat the outer surface of the tissue with india ink. This may be done either before or after specimen radiography. As an optional step, a quick dip of the inked specimen in Bouin's solution will act as a mordant and help decrease "running" of the ink during sectioning. This brief exposure to Bouin's solution will not affect receptor studies or immunohistochemistry. After blotting, the tissue can be cut in bread loaf sections at the thinnest intervals possible. If one encounters a lesion that is suggestive of invasive carcinoma, it can be handled as stated above. If there is nothing that suggests invasive carcinoma, the specimen should be fixed.

The evaluation of margins is difficult from several standpoints. Ink can run between fat cells and cleavage planes, and the inevitably irregular contour of a biopsy specimen often makes it impossible to identify the precise surgical margin. As with margins of other specimens, sampling is limited, except for the small biopsy specimens that are submitted in their entirety. Perhaps the most fundamental problem is the lack of a generally accepted determination of how close the tumor must approach an inked surface before that margin is viewed as involved. Do a few adipocytes or a narrow strand of collagen between the edge of the tumor and the surgical margin render the margin negative? Some pathologists would say yes, but others consider this narrow band of tissue to be insufficient and would view the margin as involved. There are no data to determine which approach is more clinically correct or, as Connolly and Schnitt have succinctly stated, "how close is too close." However, it is obvious that tumor clearly at an inked surface is an involved margin. When tumor cells are near, but not precisely at the inked surface, a statement regarding the distance can be made as a part of the report. Connolly and Schnitt suggest that the extent of marginal involvement, whether focal or extensive, also be a part of the report.

MAMMOGRAPHIC CALCIFICATIONS

The realization that calcium deposition is associated with carcinoma of the breast dates from 1951 (Leborgne). By the 1960s, it was recognized that radiographically detectable calcium is a major feature in the identification of nonpalpable mammary carcinomas.

Normal breast epithelium is capable of concentrating calcium for milk production. Ultrastructurally, crystalline or amorphous calcified material can be seen within the cytoplasm, either as membrane-bound or free deposits (Ahmed). The epithelial origin of calcium salts accounts for the intimate association of epithelial cells with many microcalcifications seen on tissue sections (Figures 3-1 to 3-4). Cells are often closely applied to the microcalcifications and, indeed, it is often impossible to tell whether the calcium is intracellular or extracellular. In some instances, calcium salts appear to be deposited within the cytoplasm of epithelial cells. Only when the calcium and surrounding cytoplasm are closely apposed can this be inferred (Figure 3-4). Usually, the calcium appears to lie in an extracellular location, however, because of its relatively large size (Figures 3-5, 3-6). Microcalcification adjacent to epithelium or lying free within lumina is consistent with an epithelial origin, and correlates well with the rarity of microcalcifications in the stroma. When stromal calcification is seen, it presumably has been formed by epithelium that subsequently necrosed. In our experience, stromal calcifications are usually near ducts or lobules, and it is easy to visualize how epithelium may have been previously present at those sites (Figure 3-2).

Even if calcium deposits are 100 μm or greater in diameter, as required to be visible in a mammogram, a tissue section is only about 7 μm thick. Therefore, only a small portion of a mammographically detectable calcification will appear on a tissue section. Furthermore, the majority of calcified foci in tissue sections are far less than 100 μm in diameter and, by themselves, would be invisible on a mammogram. Nevertheless, if a large number are closely approximated, they may be superimposed in sufficient volume to be detectable mammographically (Muir et al).

The correlation between the area of calcification on a mammogram and the extent of ductal carcinoma in situ is poor (Lagios et al). Gump et al described 13 patients who underwent biopsy because of microcalcification. All were treated by mastectomy, and four had residual disease not only in the biopsy site but elsewhere in the breast. The extent of the disease would not have been encompassed by a wide excision.

New deposits of mammographically detected calcium in a breast previously irradiated for invasive carcinoma are an important finding. In this clinical setting, new, noninvasive or invasive carcinoma occurs frequently. Solin et al reported that 58% of new calcifications in such patients were associated with carcinoma. This compares with the 20% to 30% yield of carcinomas in biopsy specimens containing suspicious calcifications that were removed from the general population lacking prior breast cancer.

Microcalcifications of the breast assume two major chemical forms: crystalline calcium oxalate (CaC_2O_4-$2H_2O$), and phosphate salts that are identical to hydroxyapatite ($Ca_{10}(PO_4)_6(OH)_2$). The calcium oxalate crystals are especially important, as they will not stain with H&E or a von Kossa stain. Thus, although the crystals are apparent mammographically, they may not be visible on the initial microscopic review. Only examination with polarized light will disclose them (Tornos et al and Radi). The reported discrepancy between some mammographic calcifications and the apparent absence of microcalcification in tissue sections is probably a reflection of calcium oxalate deposition.

There is a crude correlation between the two major forms of deposited calcium salts and the type of lesion with which they are associated. Calcium oxalate occurs predominately in benign breast lesions or lobular carcinoma in situ. This may reflect a very slow diffusion of calcium in a gel-type milieu (Frappart et al, 1984). Calcium phosphate is the form of calcium that is usually seen in association with ductal carcinomas, but it may also occur in benign proliferations. The calcium phosphates may precipitate on intraluminal secretory material by a mechanism that differs from that of calcium oxalate deposition (Frappart et al, 1986).

Anastassiades et al searched tissue sections for microcalcifications without regard as to whether they were radiographically detectable. There were calcifications in 19% of fibroadenomas, 26% of "fibrous disease," and 57% of fibrocystic disease. The calcifications were not found in normal breast tissue. There were granular, intracellular deposits, as well as homogeneous deposits (with and without concentric rings), mainly associated with intraluminal secreted material. Sudan stains showed that Sudan-positive material was interspersed within many of the microcalcifications. The authors believed that the proteinaceous lipid material in the microcalcifications may account for their occasionally laminated appearance (Figure 3-3).

The exact location of mammographically detected calcium in relation to abnormal tissue has been studied in a few cases. Colbassani et al carefully examined 15 cases of carcinoma, seven of which were ductal carcinoma in situ. In three cases, the calcifications were present only in the adjacent "fibrocystic disease." In nine cases, the calcifications were present only in the carcinoma. The remaining three cases had calcifications in both the carcinoma and adjacent fibrocystic disease. In 31 (78%) of 40 cases of "fibrocystic disease" the calcifications were located within the lesional tissue. In six cases (15%), it was only in the adjacent normal breast. In three cases (8%), it was present in both lesional and adjacent normal tissue. Thus, mammographically detected microcalcifications are often present within surrounding benign breast, even in biopsy specimens containing carcinoma, and the benign tissue may be the sole site of the microcalcifications (Figure 3-1).

REFERENCES

Ahmed A. Calcification in human breast carcinomas. Ultrastructural observations. *J Pathol* 1975;117:247-251.

Alberhasky MT. Mammographic and gross pathologic analysis of breast needle localization specimens. *Am J Clin Pathol* 1989;92:452-457.

Anastassiades OT, Bouropoulou V, Kontogeorgos G, et al. Microcalcifications in benign breast diseases. A histological and histochemical study. *Pathol Res Pract* 1984;178:237-242.

Bouropoulou V, Anastassiades OT, Kontogeorgos G, et al. Microcalcifications in breast carcinomas. A histological and histochemical study. *Pathol Res Pract* 1984;179:51-58.

Carter D. Margins of 'lumpectomy' for breast cancer. *Hum Pathol* 1986;17:330-332.

Colbassani HJ Jr, Feller WF, Cigtay OS, Chun B. Mammographic and pathologic correlation of microcalcification in disease of the breast. *Surg Gynecol Obstet* 1982;155:689-696.

Connolly JL, Schnitt SJ. Evaluation of breast biopsy specimens in patients considered for treatment by conservative surgery and radiation therapy for early breast cancer. *Pathol Annu* 1988;23(part 1):1-23.

Frappart I, Remy I, Lin HC, et al. Different types of microcalcifications observed in breast pathology. Correlations with histopathological diagnosis and radiological examination of operative specimens. *Virchows Arch A* 1986; 410:179-187.

Frappart L, Boudeulle M, Boumendil J, et al. Structure and composition of microcalcifications in benign and malignant lesions of the breast. Study by light microscopy, transmission and scanning electron microscopy, microprobe analysis, and x-ray diffraction. *Hum Pathol* 1984;15:880-889.

Going JJ, Anderson TJ, Crocker PR, Levison DA. Weddellite calcification in the breast. Eighteen cases with implications for breast cancer screening. *Histopathology* 1990;16:119-124.

Gump FE, Jicha DL, Ozello L. Ductal carcinoma in situ (DCIS). A revised concept. *Surgery* 1987;102:790-795.

Harris JR, Connolly JL, Schnitt SJ, et al. The use of pathologic features in selecting the extent of surgical resection necessary for breast cancer patients treated by primary radiation therapy. *Ann Surg* 1985;201:164-169.

Harris JR, Hellman S, Kinne DW. Limited surgery and radiotherapy for early breast cancer. *N Engl J Med* 1985;313:1365-1369.

Lagios ME, Westdahl PR, Margolin FR, Rose MR. Duct carcinoma *in situ*. Relationship of extent of noninvasive disease to the frequency of occult invasion, multicentricity, lymph node metastases, and short-term treatment failures. *Cancer* 1982;50:1309-1314.

Leborgne R. Diagnosis of tumors of the breast by simple roentgenography: Calcifications in carcinoma. *AJR* 1951;65:1-11.

Millis RR. Mammography. In: Azzopardi JG. *Problems in Breast Pathology*. WB Saunders Co, Philadelphia, 1979, pp 437-459.

Millis RR, Davis R, Stacey AJ. The detection and significance of calcifications in the breast. A radiological and pathological study. *Br J Radiol* 1976;49:12-26.

Muir BB, Lamb J, Anderson TJ, Kirkpatrick AE. Microcalcification and its relationship to cancer of the breast. Experience in a screening clinic. *Clin Radiol* 1983;34:193-200.

Owings D, Hann L, Schnitt SJ. How thoroughly should needle localization breast biopsies (NLBB) be sampled for microscopic examination? A prospective mammographic-pathologic correlative study. *Lab Invest* 1989;60:69A (abstract).

Patchefsky AS, Potok J, Hoch WS, Libshitz HI. Increased detection of occult breast carcinoma after more thorough histologic exami-

20   nation of breast biopsies. *Am J Clin Pathol* 1973;60:799-804.

Pope TL Jr, Fechner RE, Wilhelm MC, et al. Lobular carcinoma in situ of the breast. Mammographic features. *Radiology* 1989;168:63-66.

Radi MJ. Calcium oxalate crystals in breast biopsies. An overlooked form of microcalcification associated with benign breast disease. *Arch Pathol Lab Med* 1989;113:1367-1369.

Schnitt SJ, Wang HH. Histologic sampling of grossly benign breast biopsies. How much is enough? *Am J Surg Pathol* 1989;13:505-512.

Solin LJ, Fowble BL, Troupin RH, Goodman RL. Biopsy results of new calcifications in the postirradiated breast. *Cancer* 1989; 63: 1956-1961.

Tornos C, Silva EG, El-Naggar A, Pritzker KPH. Calcium oxalate crystals in breast biopsies. The missing microcalcifications. *Lab Invest* 1989;60:97A.

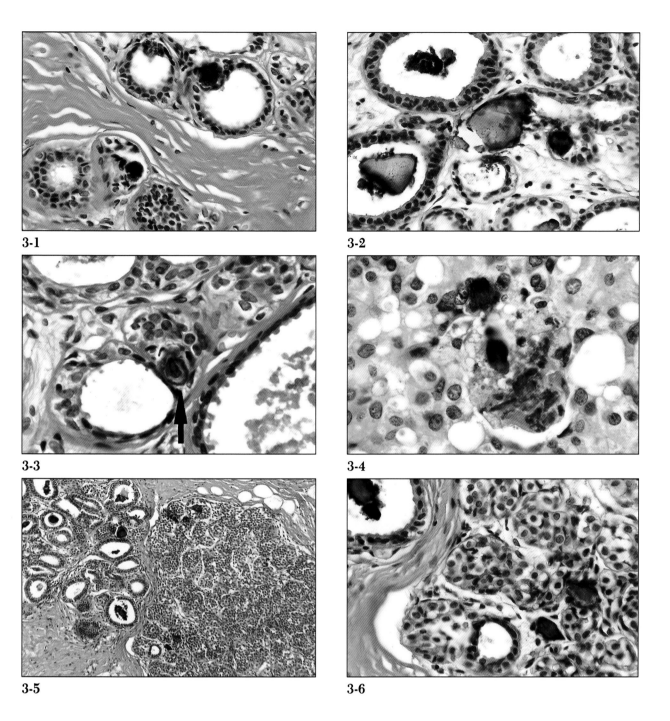

3-1

3-2

3-3

3-4

3-5

3-6

Figure 3-1. Normal lobules may contain calcium deposits. In one ductule, the epithelium on the luminal side appears stretched over the calcium deposit (upper right). In the other ductule, the calcium appears to be free-floating, but is associated with discohesive cells that may be undergoing necrosis after depositing the calcium.

Figure 3-3. Occasionally, calcium deposits have a laminated configuration, with sequential layers of deposition evident.

Figure 3-5. A large area of lobular carcinoma in situ contains a few calcifications (right). The calcifications are also in an uninvolved lobule (left).

Figure 3-2. The largest deposit of calcium has been partly fractured by tissue sectioning. It lies partially within the stroma, although epithelial cells are in continuity. Uneven staining of the calcium is seen.

Figure 3-4. A comedocarcinoma contains irregularly shaped deposits of calcium in intimate association with the cytoplasm of apparently degenerating neoplastic cells. It is likely that some of the smaller intracytoplasmic basophilic deposits are calcium salts.

Figure 3-6. Higher magnification of Figure 3-5 discloses apparent stromal calcium (lower right). Intraluminal calcification that may represent calcified secretory material is seen in the nonneoplastic ductule at upper left.

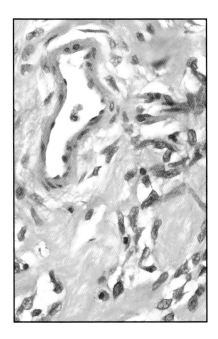

4

Vascular and Pseudovascular Changes

Clinically important vascular tumors of the breast are rare. When confronted with a vascular or vascular-like proliferation in this location, the critical distinction is between angiosarcoma and a variety of benign lesions. Before discussing the latter group, it is appropriate to define the criteria for the diagnosis of angiosarcoma. Several studies have indicated that grading mammary angiosarcomas correlates with prognosis (Donnell et al, Merino et al, Rosen et al). However, angiosarcomas may show marked variability in their microscopic appearance, with a tendency for low-grade areas to be located peripherally (Donnell et al). Therefore, grading is most applicable to well-sampled, complete resections.

High-grade angiosarcomas are readily recognized by their prominent cellularity, conspicuous nuclear pleomorphism, and numerous mitotic figures, coupled with tufting of the endothelial cells and papillary proliferations. High-grade lesions also have solid, nonvascular areas composed of malignant spindle cells. Necrosis and "blood lakes" are almost always present. Intermediate-grade angiosarcomas have focal endothelial tufting, focal papillary proliferations, and minimal or absent solid spindle cell foci. They lack necrosis or blood lakes.

Low-grade angiosarcoma is more likely to be confused with a benign vascular lesion than with the overtly malignant high-grade lesions. Although low-grade angiosarcomas often have small, hyperchromatic nuclei, cytologic criteria are not particularly helpful, given the overlap of the mild cytologic abnormalities in low-grade angiosarcoma with those of some benign vascular or pseudovascular tumors. The diagnosis of low-grade angiosarcoma is made predominantly on the irregular branching (anastomosing) pattern of the vessels (Figures 4-1, 4-2). The vessels invade fat, surround ducts, and may infiltrate the stroma within lobules. However, this infiltrating pattern is not pathognomonic of angiosarcoma, as it also occurs in some benign vascular and pseudovascular lesions. Another distinctive feature of angiosarcoma is the highly variable distribution of vessels, which may be numerous in some areas and widely separated by fat or fibrous tissue in other foci.

PSEUDOANGIOMATOUS CHANGE AND HYPERPLASIA

Pseudoangiomatous change is seen in about 20% of all breast biopsy specimens (Ibrahim et al). The area of involvement usually covers no more than a few low-power fields and is not detectable on gross examination. In this process the stromal fibrous tissue is intermixed with spindle cells. The latter line empty spaces, and the spaces are separated from one another by dense, sparsely cellular collagen (Figures 4-3, 4-4). The anastomosing pattern of the spaces, coupled with their flat lining cells, imparts a vascular appearance to the tissue. Mitotic figures are sometimes seen in the stromal cells, adding to the confusion with a vascular proliferation (Figure 4-5). The spaces are devoid of blood, however, and immunohistochemical, as well as ultrastructural, studies confirm that the spindle cells are fibroblasts, not endothelial cells. True capillaries are, of course widely scattered among the pseudoangiomatous channels (Figure 4-6). Small foci of this distinctive stromal alteration may develop without apparent stromal proliferation, so that ducts and lobules are preserved in what appears to be their original relationship.

Rarely, pseudoangiomatous change may be associated with stromal hyperplasia (pseudoangiomatous hyperplasia) that results in a clinically palpable mass 2 to 7 cm in diameter. These masses are tan or gray and well demarcated. Dilated ducts may be visible as cysts of varying size on cut surfaces. About a dozen clinically palpable cases have been reported; all were in premenopausal women ranging from 21 to 52 years of age. A few patients have had local recurrences. The pathogenesis and long-term implications of this process are unknown.

HEMANGIOMAS AND PERILOBULAR HEMANGIOMAS

Mammary hemangiomas are common incidental findings. Lesueur et al detected them in 11% of breasts. A few lesions were 3 to 4 mm in size, but most were smaller than 1.5 mm. Occasionally, they were multiple or bilateral. The most common location for small mammary hemangiomas is in areas adjacent to lobules. These so-called perilobular hemangiomas are usually well circumscribed, but some capillaries may extend into the adjacent fat or fibrous stroma, or between the ductules of the lobule. Regardless of their local extension, the capillaries are usually of uniform size and lack the anastomosing pattern of angiosarcoma (Figures 4-7, 4-8). The endothelial cell nuclei of perilobular hemangioma may be slightly enlarged and ovoid to round, and may bulge into the capillary lumen (Figures 4-9, 4-10).

Jozefczyk and Rosen described a group of atypical hemangiomas that had mild cytologic abnormalities and focal anastomosis of vascular channels. The lesions occurred in women between the ages of 43 and 71 years, with most patients over the age of 60 years. Some were incidental microscopic findings, whereas others were palpable or identified on mammogram. With one exception, the atypical hemangiomas were sharply circumscribed, although septation sometimes resulted in ill-defined lobules. The endothelial cells had enlarged, rounded nuclei and a mild degree of pleomorphism. Most of the lesions had vessels of capillary size, but some had a cavernous component. A spindle cell component, presumably stromal, was seen focally. Although follow-up is limited, patients treated with local excision have not developed a recurrence.

ANGIOMATOSIS

Angiomatosis of the breast is, fortunately, extremely rare. It is especially likely to be misdiagnosed as angiosarcoma because of its irregular, variably sized, anastomosing vessels that extend between ductal structures, lobules, and fat (Figure 4-11). Angiomatosis does not produce a circumscribed mass, and simple mastectomy may be required to remove large, diffuse lesions (Rosen, Morrow et al). Incomplete excision may lead to recurrence. Distinction from angiosarcoma requires multiple sections from a complete excision specimen. Unlike low-grade angiosarcoma, the vessels of angiomatosis tend to be evenly distributed and lack the tendency to diminish in size at the periphery of the lesion. Intralobular growth is not as common in angiomatosis as in angiosarcoma. The endothelial nuclei of angiomatosis are small and often rather difficult to detect, and papillary tufting is absent (Figure 4-12).

MISCELLANEOUS VASCULAR LESIONS

Venous hemangiomas have been reported in four patients. The large, irregular vascular channels in these lesions resembled a cavernous hemangioma of soft tissues and had varying amounts of smooth muscle in their walls. As with angiomatosis, breast parenchyma was interspersed among the vascular channels. Distinction from low-grade angiosarcoma was based on the absence of nuclear pleomorphism, nuclear hyperchromasia, papillary tufting or hyperplasia, mitotic figures, necrosis, or destructive invasion. Also helpful are the presence of smooth muscle in the vessel walls and the overall circumscription of the lesion (Rosen et al, 1985).

Hemangiopericytomas located within the substance of the breast are rare. Thus far, they have been pathologically low grade, although some may be large (Tavassoli and Weiss). The subcutaneous tissue of the breast also may be the site of cavernous hemangiomas, juvenile hemangiomas, lobular capillary hemangiomas, papillary endothelial hyperplasia, and angiolipomas. The differential diagnosis of these lesions is the same as when they occur in the soft tissues of other sites.

REFERENCES

Arias-Stella J Jr, Rosen PP. Hemangiopericytoma of the breast. *Mod Pathol* 1988;1:98-103.

Donnell RM, Rosen PP, Lieberman PH, et al. Angiosarcoma and other vascular tumors of the breast. Pathologic analysis as a guide to prognosis. *Am J Surg Pathol* 1981;5:629-642.

Ibrahim RE, Sciotto CG, Weidner N. Pseudoangiomatous hyperplasia of mammary stroma. Some observations regarding its clinicopathologic spectrum. *Cancer* 1989; 63: 1154-1160.

Jozefczyk MA, Rosen PP. Vascular tumors of the breast. II. Perilobular hemangiomas and hemangiomas. *Am J Surg Pathol* 1985;9:491-503.

Lesueur GC, Brown RW, Bhathal PS. Incidence of perilobular hemangioma in the female breast. *Arch Pathol Lab Med* 1983;107:308-310.

Merino MJ, Carter D, Berman M. Angiosarcoma of the breast. *Am J Surg Pathol* 1983;7:53-60.

Morrow M, Berger D, Thelmo W. Diffuse cystic angiomatosis of the breast. *Cancer* 1988;62:2392-2396.

Rosen PP. Vascular tumors of the breast. III. Angiomatosis. *Am J Surg Pathol* 1985; 9: 652-658.

Rosen PP, Jozefczyk MA, Boram LH. Vascular tumors of the breast. IV. The venous hemangioma. *Am J Surg Pathol* 1985;9:659-665.

Rosen PP. Vascular tumors of the breast. V. Nonparenchymal hemangiomas of mammary subcutaneous tissues. *Am J Surg Pathol* 1985;9:723-729.

Rosen PP, Kimmel M, Ernsberger D. Mammary angiosarcoma. The prognostic significance of tumor differentiation. *Cancer* 1988;62:2145-2151.

Tavassoli FA, Weiss S. Hemangiopericytoma of the breast. *Am J Surg Pathol* 1981;5:745-752.

Vuitch MF, Rosen PP, Erlandson RA. Pseudoangiomatous hyperplasia of mammary stroma. *Hum Pathol* 1986;17:185-191.

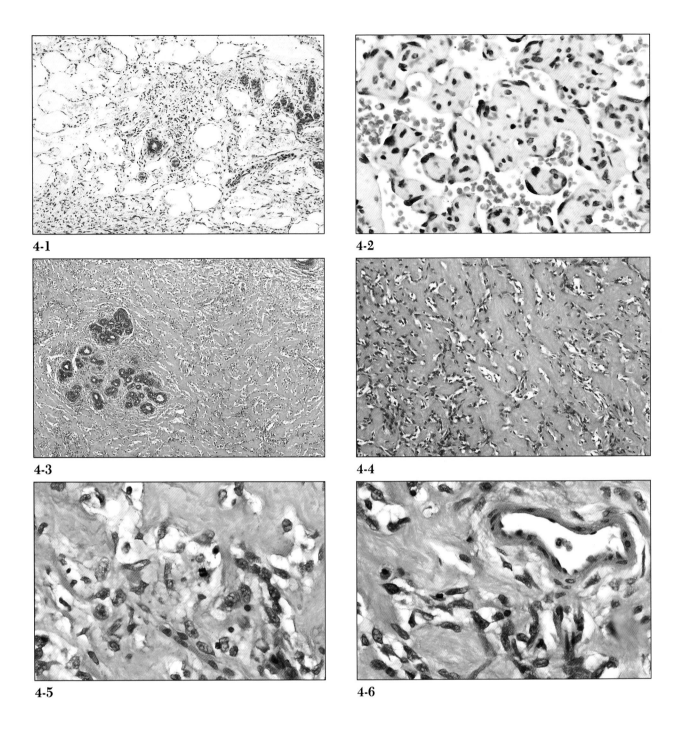

4-1

4-2

4-3

4-4

4-5

4-6

Figure 4-1. The irregular branching and anastomosing vessels seen here typify low-grade angiosarcoma. Note that individual ductules are isolated by the proliferating vascular channels.

Figure 4-3. Pseudoangiomatous hyperplasia surrounds lobules. Clefts are prominent, imparting an infiltrating, vascular-like appearance.

Figure 4-5. Stromal cells in the pseudovascular clefts may show nuclear enlargement and, rarely, mitotic activity. Numerous delicate cytoplasmic strands bridge the bloodless clefts.

Figure 4-2. At higher magnification, low-grade angiosarcoma exhibits mild but definite nuclear pleomorphism. Anastomosing vascular channels are clearly seen.

Figure 4-4. The pseudovascular clefts are irregularly spaced between dense, hypocellular collagen bundles.

Figure 4-6. The cells of pseudoangiomatous hyperplasia are larger than normal endothelial cells. Again, note the lack of erythrocytes and presence of cytoplasmic strands in the cleft-like spaces.

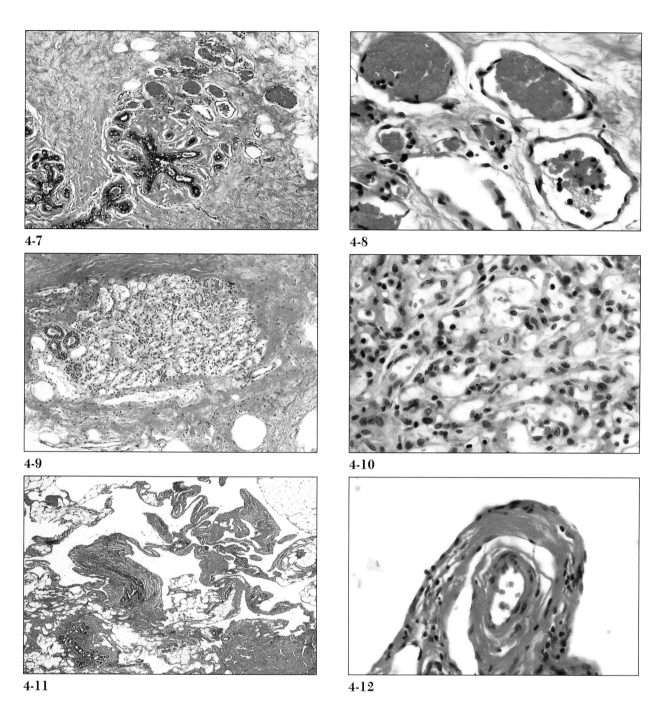

4-7

4-8

4-9

4-10

4-11

4-12

Figure 4-7. Perilobular hemangioma usually consists of similarly sized, nonanastomosing capillaries closely associated with a lobule.

Figure 4-9. Perilobular hemangiomas may consist of smaller, more closely approximated capillaries. The sharp circumscription and lack of anastomosing channels allow distinction from angiosarcoma.

Figure 4-11. Angiomatosis is characterized by large, anastomosing vessels that extend between ducts and lobules, and infiltrate adipose tissue. A variable amount of smooth muscle is present in the vessel walls.

Figure 4-8. The capillaries of perilobular hemangioma are lined by normal endothelial cells.

Figure 4-10. The nuclei of the perilobular hemangioma seen in Figure 4-9 are slightly enlarged and ovoid, but they lack the hyperchromasia of low-grade angiosarcoma.

Figure 4-12. Both the large sinusoid at the top of the field and the central capillary are lined by small, normal-appearing endothelial cells.

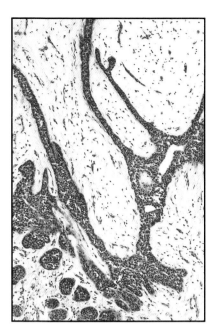

5

FIBROADENOMAS, ADENOMAS, AND HAMARTOMAS

Several rather common palpable or mammographically detectable lesions in the breast are characterized, microscopically, by a proliferation of glandular elements and varying amounts of stroma. The fibroadenoma is the prototypical member of this group. More recently, other related benign epithelial or epithelial and stromal proliferations have been described using such terms as *adenoma* and *hamartoma*. As will be discussed in this section, the diagnostic criteria for some of these latter lesions are not as well established as for fibroadenoma.

FIBROADENOMA

Fibroadenoma (adenofibroma) of the breast is a common, benign tumor composed of fibrous and epithelial elements. Although adjectives such as "intracanalicular" and "pericanalicular" have been used to subtype fibroadenomas, they are of no practical importance and merely identify variations in the arrangement of the stroma and epithelium. Other modifiers applied to fibroadenoma such as "giant" and "juvenile" are of more importance, predominantly because of their inconsistent usage. For example, giant fibroadenoma has been used interchangeably with "benign cystosarcoma phyllodes." As is discussed below, the histologic features of these two lesions differ and their similar size is irrelevant. Juvenile fibroadenoma, if properly defined, has a constellation of clinical and pathologic features that separate it from the ordinary adult-type fibroadenoma, whether or not the latter occurs in young girls. Adult and juvenile fibroadenomas will be discussed separately.

Adult Fibroadenoma

An adult–type fibroadenoma is a sharply circumscribed proliferation of epithelium and stroma. It originates from the terminal duct-lobular unit and may be as small as the diameter of three or four lobules. At the other extreme is the giant fibroadenoma. Although there is no defined minimal size, this term probably should be reserved for lesions greater than 8 to 10 cm in diameter or weighing at least 500 g. Occasional giant fibroadenomas may measure up to 20 cm in diameter. Approximately half of fibroadenomas occur in women between the ages of 20 and 35 years, and most of the remainder arise in women between 35 and 45 years of age. About 10% occur in teenagers and an equal number develop in patients over 45 years of age. Many of the lesions seen in postmenopausal women are mammographic findings rather than palpable tumors. Frantz et al found a 9% prevalence of fibroadenomas in an autopsy study of clinically normal breasts. Most of these lesions were microscopic, and only 2% were grossly visible.

Fibroadenomas that are observed clinically usually double in size during the first 6 to 12 months (Haagensen), and often cease growing when they reach 2 to 3 cm in diameter. Ten percent to 20% of fibroadenomas are synchronously multiple. They may be concentrated in one quadrant of the breast or dispersed in several quadrants. About 3% are bilateral, and the frequency of new lesions is about 5%. There is a tendency for new lesions to occur in the ipsilateral breast, although with the specific clinical exception noted below, patients with bilateral, synchronous tumors do not have an overall increased risk for recurrence (Oliver and Major).

One clinically distinct subgroup of patients with fibroadenomas consists of black females with multiple, usually bilateral fibroadenomas that occur in successive "waves" of recurrent lesions (Oberman). The subsequent tumors appear within a few months to several years after surgery. These lesions are histologically indistinguishable from typical adult-type fibroadenomas.

Fibroadenomas have a rather consistent gross appearance. Typically, they form a sharply delineated, spherical or discoid mass that has a white cut surface. Occasionally, there may be light brown areas corresponding to a prominent epithelial component. Small clefts may be visible and these can be accentuated by slightly bending the cut surface. Most fibroadenomas are firm but not hard, except for some lesions with densely collagenized, focally calcified stroma that occur in elderly patients. A few fibroadenomas in elderly women are indistinguishable grossly and microscopically from those in young patients.

Microscopically, the fibrous stroma is the most prominent and variable component of fibroadenomas. The stroma can compress and distort ductules or small ducts, reducing them to small, curvilinear slits (intracanalicular pattern) (Figure 5-1). In other areas, the ducts may maintain their patency and circular shape because the stroma grows circumferentially around them (pericanalicular pattern). Mixtures of intracanalicular and pericanalicular patterns are common.

The adult-type fibroadenoma may have the normal double layer of cells, or it may exhibit proliferative changes ranging from epithelial tufting to more florid hyperplasia (Figures 5-2 to 5-4). The latter may be ex-aggerated by tangential sectioning of irregular ducts. The cytologic appearance of the hyperplastic cells is the same as is described and illustrated in the section on hyperplasia in fibrocystic change (see page 92). Approximately 14% of fibroadenomas will have small foci of apocrine metaplasia (Figure 5-5). Squamous metaplasia with or without keratinization is rare. Mitotic figures are occasionally numerous, but always have a normal configuration. Well-formed lobules are frequently maintained in fibroadenomas, and during pregnancy these lobules may show lactational change. This change has also been reported in women using oral contraceptives (Figure 5-6). Fibroadenomas from the latter women, however, do not have other alterations such as epithelial atypia. Azzopardi found sclerosing adenosis in 6% of fibroadenomas, especially in tumors from older patients. This is not surprising given the lobular origin of both lesions (Figures 5-7, 5-8).

Approximately one in 200 fibroadenomas is partially or totally infarcted. About one half of women with infarction have pain or tenderness, and most are pregnant or lactating. Occasionally, a thrombosed, medium-sized artery is identifiable.

The cellularity of the stroma in fibroadenomas varies greatly, as does the amount of collagen. Myxoid areas may be especially paucicellular. Other foci may be cellular with a modest degree of pleomorphism. Mitotic figures may be numerous, with as many as two or three mitotic figures per ten high-power fields. Fibroadenomas may also contain densely cellular areas and, when coupled with a high mitotic rate or atypical cells, these regions raise the possibility of phyllodes tumor (see below).

Fibroadenomas may contain variable amounts of fat. This probably represents entrapment, as fibroadenomas grow, at least in part, by incorporating lobules at their periphery. Osseous and smooth muscle metaplasia are seen rarely. When the latter component is very prominent, the term *muscular hamartoma* has been used. This term has also been applied to those masses that are almost exclusively smooth muscle and lack the epithelial features of fibroadenoma (Huntrakoon and Lin).

Rarely, the stroma of a fibroadenoma contains haphazardly scattered multinucleated giant cells that can have anywhere from a few to numerous nuclei (Figures 5-9, 5-10). The latter are often closely clustered, or they may have a floret pattern. The multinucleated cells were shown by Berean et al to be of fibroblastic origin. Fibroadenomas with multinucleated giant cells do not have other features of phyllodes tumor such as a highly cellular stroma or increased mitotic activity. Moreover, multinucleated giant cells are not typical in phyllodes tumor (Figures 5-11, 5-12).

Differential Diagnosis. The differential diagnosis of fibroadenomas includes lesions that have either abnormal epithelium, abnormal stroma, or both. Most, if not all carcinomas arising in fibroadenomas have occurred in the adult-type variant. Because of this association, the phenomenon of carcinoma arising in fibroadenoma is discussed below in this section. The phyllodes tumor is most often confused with juvenile fibroadenoma, and this distinction is discussed under the latter heading.

By 1985, about 100 cases of either noninvasive or invasive carcinoma arising in fibroadenomas had been reported (Figures 5-13 to 5-18). Approximately one half of the carcinomas have been lobular carcinoma in situ, 35% have been infiltrating carcinoma (either infiltrating lobular or infiltrating ductal), and 15% have been ductal carcinoma in situ. In one series, carcinoma was found in two of 73 fibroadenomas removed from women between the ages of 40 and 60 (Deschênes et al). About 40% of patients with carcinoma in a fibroadenoma have carcinoma in the breast tissue adjacent to the nodule (Pick and Iossifides). Carcinomas arising in fibroadenomas do not seem to differ, biologically, from the corresponding form of carcinoma arising de novo. For example, some patients with lobular carcinoma in situ in a fibroadenoma have had long-term disease-free intervals without further therapy, whereas others have subsequently developed invasive carcinomas, either in the ipsilateral or contralateral breast (Ozzello and Gump).

Traditionally, patients with fibroadenomas have not been considered to have an increased frequency of subsequent carcinoma, but recent data suggest such an increased risk (DuPont et al). Kodlin et al found that 16 of 849 women with fibroadenomas developed carcinoma, whereas 2.3 were statistically predicted to develop cancer, based on incidence rates for the general population. This increased risk is similar to that described by Moskowitz et al, who studied a selected group of perimenopausal and postmenopausal women with fibroadenomas who had voluntarily entered a breast cancer detection center.

Fibromatosis of the breast may mimic fibroadenoma because the proliferating fibrous tissue in the former lesion surrounds ducts and lobules, incorporating them into a mass that may be several centimeters wide (Ali et al). In general, fibromatosis is much more cellular than the stroma of fibroadenoma, but, most importantly, it has an infiltrating margin. Fibrous tissue at the margins of fibromatosis extends between fat cells, whereas the fibrous tissue at the periphery of fibroadenomas abuts but does not infiltrate the surrounding stroma. It should be noted that although fibroadenomas are sharply circumscribed, contrary to frequent statements, they are usually unencapsulated.

Juvenile Fibroadenoma

Juvenile fibroadenoma is an accepted term for a histologically distinctive fibroadenoma variant that occurs mainly in teenagers. It makes up approximately 4% of fibroadenomas (Fekete et al). In the past, this lesion has been included in the categories of benign phyllodes tumor, giant fibroadenoma, and cellular fibroadenoma. The term juvenile fibroadenoma reflects the almost exclusive occurrence in teenagers who are usually 1 to 3 years postmenarche or, occasionally, premenarche. Blacks are more often afflicted than whites. Lesions with the microscopic features of juvenile fibroadenoma can also occur in women between 20 and 40 years of age. Tumors in older patients have been referred to as fibroadenomas with stromal cellularity to avoid the semantically inaccurate term of "juvenile." Mies and Rosen found fibroadenomas with hypercellular stroma and epithelium in a few women beyond the age of 50 years, the oldest being 72 years of age.

The clinical manifestations of juvenile fibroadenomas fall into two major groups. In one group the tumor appears as a solitary mass, and these patients rarely develop an additional tumor. The other group is characterized by multiple tumors, usually in both breasts. After surgical removal of these tumors, almost all patients in the latter group develop recurrences within 12 to 18 months. There may be additional recurrences, although they typically become less frequent as the patients enter adulthood. Moreover, in the group with multiple recurrences, some lesions that are left in place cease to grow. In many patients with single tumors, there is rapid growth for a few months that enlarges the affected breast to two or more times the size of its unaffected counterpart. The skin is often stretched and the nipple displaced, and there may be dilatation of superficial veins.

Mies and Rosen noted two patients who developed noninvasive carcinomas 5 and 19 years after excision of a juvenile fibroadenoma. Whether or not an increased risk for subsequent carcinoma exists will depend on the accumulation of many more cases coupled with long-term follow-up.

The gross appearance of juvenile fibroadenomas is often indistinguishable from fibroadenomas of the usual type, as described above. Some juvenile fibroadenomas, however, are more nodular and may have irregular areas that are pink or tan. This variegated appearance is more common in large, rapidly enlarging lesions. Juvenile fibroadenomas can range from 2 to 22 cm in size. In one series, the median diameter for solitary lesions was 2.8 cm, and for multiple lesions it was 2.2 cm (Fekete et al).

The microscopic spectrum is broad. Nonetheless, there is a definite trend toward greater stromal cellularity and more epithelial hyperplasia than in the usual adult-type lesion. In approximately half of juvenile fibroadenomas the epithelial component consists of well-formed lobules. These are usually distorted by the intervening stromal proliferation. Enlarged ductules are usually numerous and may contain hyperplastic epithelium four to eight cells thick (Figures 5-19, 5-20) with superimposed small papillations. The papillary tufts often have cells containing less cytoplasm than those in the intramural epithelial component, imparting an appearance identical to the proliferative form of gynecomastia (Figure 5-19). The epithelium may also assume a more complex bridging pattern with interconnecting loops of cells (Figures 5-21, 5-22). The same variation in nuclei that is seen in typical hyperplasia of fibrocystic change is present. Nuclei normally vary in their density, often overlap, and are irregularly distributed. Mild nuclear atypia may occasionally be seen (Figure 5-23). There are scattered mitotic figures, but necrosis is not evident.

The stroma is focally or diffusely hypercellular with considerable pleomorphism (Figure 5-24). Mitotic figures in stromal cells are found in 30% to 40% of cases. Usually, there are fewer than three mitotic figures per ten high-power (X 400) fields, but slightly higher mitotic rates have been observed. Regardless of the mitotic count, none of the sol-

itary tumors has recurred. Although most of the stroma is hypercellular, there may be large areas that are sparsely cellular and heavily collagenized. Multinucleated stromal giant cells may be present occasionally, but, unlike adult-type fibroadenomas, myxoid stroma is rare.

Differential Diagnosis—Diffuse (Virginal) Hypertrophy. The differential diagnosis of juvenile fibroadenoma includes diffuse (virginal) hypertrophy of the breast. The latter process usually produces diffuse and massive, symmetric, bilateral enlargement. Clinically, the rapid enlargement and flattening of the nipple are similar to the changes seen with a giant juvenile fibroadenoma. Microscopically, there may be focal areas that have the stromal and epithelial alterations of juvenile fibroadenoma. However, diffuse hypertrophy is dominated by connective tissue with minimal or absent lobule formation. In one patient described by Oberman there was enlargement of residual breast tissue 7 months after a reduction mammoplasty had been done for diffuse hypertrophy.

Differential Diagnosis—Phyllodes Tumor. The adult and juvenile variants of fibroadenoma must be distinguished histologically from phyllodes tumor. Size is not a criterion for this distinction because, as previously discussed, some fibroadenomas may be quite large. The term *giant fibroadenoma*, as applied to the latter lesions, should not be used interchangeably with the semantically abominable term *benign cystosarcoma phyllodes*. A giant fibroadenoma is nothing more than a microscopically conventional fibroadenoma that has attained a large size.

We and many others prefer the term *phyllodes tumor*, as suggested by the World Health Organization, rather than the older term of cystosarcoma phyllodes. Phyllodes tumor may be easily modified, as appropriate, with the prefixes benign, borderline, or malignant. This avoids the seemingly irrational designation of benign cystosarcoma phyllodes.

Our criteria for the diagnosis of phyllodes tumor require an extremely hypercellular stroma with numerous foci of irregular intracanalicular growth (Figures 5-11, 5-12). This is coupled with large, dilated ducts that have irregular configurations due to the stromal proliferation. *Phyllodes* is the Greek word for leaf and refers to the leaf-like patterns of the irregular stromal protrusions into the dilated ducts. The stromal hypercellularity may be clustered beneath the epithelium, or there may be a hypocellular, subepithelial zone with the hypercellular areas located between the ducts.

Phyllodes tumor may have sparsely cellular, hyalinized areas or myxoid stroma. In such instances one must concentrate on the most cellular foci to differentiate benign (ie, nonmetastasizing) from malignant forms. Phyllodes tumors with numerous bizarre nuclei and mitotic rates exceeding five per ten high-power fields pose no problem and are readily recognized as malignant. Stromal overgrowth, defined as one low-power field of stroma lacking epithelium, is also a highly suggestive feature of malignancy. This change is not seen in all lesions classified as malignant phyllodes tumor, but it is especially important to recognize, as most tumors that metastasize have this feature. Areas resembling fibrosarcoma, liposarcoma, chondrosarcoma, osteosarcoma, or rhabdomyosarcoma also indicate malignancy.

The epithelial elements of phyllodes tumor are not distinctive when compared with fibroadenoma. The ducts may be lined by a two-cell population, or have ductal hyperplasia of the usual type. There may be squamous metaplasia, as well as foci of sclerosing adenosis. As with fibroadenomas, a concurrent lobular or ductal carcinoma in situ may be present.

Phyllodes tumor is uncommon in women younger than 30 years of age. Of the 26 patients described by Ward and Evans, only three (15, 25, and 28 years of age) were under 30 years of age. Thus, the giant fibroadenoma, which is usually seen in teenagers or women in their early 20s, occurs in an age group in which phyllodes tumor is uncommon. Rare cases of so-called periductal fibrosarcoma have been described in teenagers. Pike and Oberman reported an example in a 17-year-old, and Adami et al reported another in a 16-year-old. In reality, these appear to be extraordinarily rare examples of malignant phyllodes tumor in adolescents.

TUBULAR ADENOMA AND LACTATING ADENOMA

In 1968, Persaud and colleagues emphasized the rarity of true mammary adenomas and accepted reports of only two cases from the literature. They believed that most so-called ad-

enomas were actually fibroadenomas with a greater than usual lobular component.

Tubular Adenoma

Tubular adenoma is best defined as a circumscribed mass consisting of closely packed ductules with little intervening stroma. Women with tubular adenomas range from 16 to 40 years of age, although most are in their third decade of life. Not unexpectedly in this age group, there is often a history of oral contraceptive use, but there is no evidence that this is causative. Women with tubular adenomas may have a typical fibroadenoma, either in the same or the opposite breast. On occasion, the adenoma may abut the fibroadenoma (Hertel et al).

Tubular adenomas of the breast have been associated with malignancy in only two instances. Hill and Miller described a 34-year-old woman who had an adenoma that was microscopically involved with carcinoma. She had widespread cancer, and no mastectomy was performed. It seems highly likely that the adenoma was secondarily invaded by the carcinoma. One other report by Case is not sufficiently documented to be certain of the adenoma-to-carcinoma relationship.

Tubular adenomas range from 0.8 to 4 cm in diameter, but most are between 1.5 and 3.0 cm. These are sharply circumscribed (Figure 5-25) and firm but not hard. The cut surface is yellow or tan and may be finely nodular. Microscopically, tubular adenomas are usually sharply demarcated, but rarely are encapsulated. An irregular margin of proliferating ductules occasionally extends into the surrounding fat (Figure 5-26). The ductules of tubular adenoma are indistinguishable from those of normal breast (Figures 5-27, 5-28). There is no nuclear atypia, and mitotic figures are rare. Tubular adenomas may be infarcted, especially in women who are pregnant or lactating.

Differential Diagnosis. The differential diagnosis of tubular adenoma includes fibroadenoma and tubular carcinoma. Most fibroadenomas have an obvious stromal component, but a few will have predominant epithelial elements and, in occasional cases, may approach the appearance of a tubular adenoma. Tubular adenomas are distinguished by their lack of elongated ducts and the presence of only a minimal, nonneoplastic supporting stroma. Lesions with more than this minimal

34

stroma should be labeled as fibroadenomas to maintain the homogeneity of the tubular adenoma category. Obviously, this distinction currently has little or no clinical importance.

Avoiding confusion of tubular adenoma with tubular carcinoma is of considerable clinical importance, and this distinction is readily made, both on gross and microscopic grounds. Tubular carcinoma feels hard on palpation and has a white cut surface with a stellate configuration identical to that of infiltrating ductal carcinoma. Microscopically, the neoplastic tubules are lined by a solitary layer of cuboidal epithelium that is almost completely devoid of a myoepithelial component at the light microscopic level. Tubular carcinoma elicits a desmoplastic reaction that surrounds almost every tubule. This stromal response is more cellular and heavily collagenized than the delicate stroma of tubular adenoma. In addition, the stromal response results in much more widely dispersed tubules than in tubular adenoma.

Lactating Adenoma

The existence of lactating adenoma as a distinct entity has been questioned. The term can be used for a circumscribed mass consisting of closely approximated ductules with secretory activity. There are several hypotheses to explain lactating adenoma as just defined. O'Hara and Page noted histologic similarities between lactating adenomas and fibroadenomas with lactational changes. They suggested that lactating adenomas might arise in preexisting fibroadenomas. It seems unlikely, however, that this hypothesis explains all lactating adenomas. The fibrous component of a fibroadenoma is maintained during pregnancy or lactation, even when there is conspicuous secretory activity and an accentuated lobular proliferation (LeGal). It is more likely that at least some lactating adenomas arise in preexisting tubular adenomas as a physiological response to pregnancy. An alternative explanation is that lactating adenomas are merely areas of pregnancy/lactation-induced lobular proliferation that are more prominent than in the remainder of the breast. This would reflect the physiological variability that is so characteristic of mammary parenchyma. Finally, it is possible that some lactating adenomas are true benign neoplasms arising de novo during pregnancy.

Lactating adenomas vary from 1 to 4 cm in diameter. They are tan or slightly yellow, sharply demarcated nodules. A lobulated appearance is often conspicuous. Because of their secretory activity, they tend to be softer than tubular adenomas and may exude a milky substance when sectioned.

Microscopically, lactating adenomas form true acini identical to those seen in normal lactating breast (Figure 5-29). The acini are populated by cells with enlarged nuclei and copious, vacuolated cytoplasm (Figure 5-30). Hertel et al noted that the lactating adenomas excised in the first 6 months of pregnancy had more stroma than those excised after that time. This observation provides some support for the altered fibroadenoma theory for the origin of lactating adenoma as described above.

SCLEROSING LOBULAR HYPERPLASIA

Sclerosing lobular hyperplasia is a mass characterized by hyperplasia of the lobules with intervening fibrosis. The term reflects an increase in both the number of ductules per lobule and the total number of lobules in a given volume of tissue. Patients range from 14 to 41 years of age, with a peak incidence between 26 and 35 years. Sclerosing lobular hyperplasia presents as a painless or slightly tender mass, usually of 1 or 2 months' duration. In the study by Kovi et al, all of the patients were black, but because their overall patient population was almost exclusively black, no conclusions can be drawn about racial predisposition. We have seen the same lesion in white patients.

On gross inspection, the mass is usually sharply circumscribed but without a capsule. The cut surface discloses irregularly shaped, tan nodules representing large lobules. Microscopically, the lobular architecture is maintained (Figures 5-31, 5-32), with the enlarged lobules composed of increased numbers of individually normal ductules (Figure 5-33). Sclerosing lobular hyperplasia may be associated with fibroadenomas. Conversely, almost half of the patients reported by Kovi et al to have fibroadenomas had adjacent foci of sclerosing lobular hyperplasia. Moreover, some of the latter foci contained a more prominent stroma with distortion of the ducts, characterized as "incipient" fibroadenoma formation.

HAMARTOMA

Hamartoma and adenolipoma are terms that have been given to a pathologically heterogeneous group of benign lesions presenting as discrete round or discoid masses. Review of the literature shows that these terms have been applied to overlapping microscopic images. We agree with Linell et al that "there is good reason to believe that there is a continuous variation from fibrous and glandular hamartomas to typical adenolipomas."

In some publications, the young age of the patients and the microscopic descriptions suggest that the lesions called hamartoma might now be better classified as juvenile fibroadenomas. For example, case 10 reported by Linell et al was considered a hamartoma, although the mass appeared 2 to 3 years after menarche and grew rapidly to double the volume of the opposite breast. Similarly, we believe that another case diagnosed as hamartoma is actually a fibroadenoma (Petrik).

It must be recognized that there are sharply circumscribed, benign masses in the breast that simply do not fit within current classification schemes. This is not an admission of diagnostic failure, but an acknowledgement of the broadly diverse images that varying proportions of epithelial and stromal proliferations can produce.

Mammary hamartomas have occurred in women from 15 to 88 years of age, with the majority of patients being beyond the age of 35 years. The mean ages in four series ranged from 38 to 45 years (Arrigoni et al, Hessler et al, Linell et al, Oberman). Hamartomas are unilateral, and recurrence has not been reported. Some women have had the masses detected after lactation. There may still be secretory changes in the lobules, but the predominance of fibrous tissue distinguishes such lesions from lactating adenomas. Other patients have been nulliparous, indicating that hamartoma is not necessarily a residuum of previously lactating breast.

There does not appear to be an association with other breast diseases. The reported follow-up of women with hamartomas has been short, but none has developed carcinoma. Hessler et al found hamartomas in 16 of 10,000 consecutive mammograms. Hamartomas are considered to be mammographically distinctive, and the lesion need not be removed if the diagnosis is radiographically secure.

Lesions designated as hamartomas of the breast have ranged from 1 to 17 cm in diameter, but most are 2 to 4 cm in diameter. Their consistency is less firm than that of fibroadenomas. They are not encapsulated, but are sharply circumscribed (Figure 5-34). The microscopic variation in the stroma and epithelium of hamartomas was emphasized by Arrigoni et al. The amount of fibrous tissue varies, and some lesions classified as hamartomas have consisted mainly of fibrous tissue with only a few ductal or lobular elements. The fibrous tissue may be densely collagenous and sparsely cellular or prominently cellular with loose collagen. Fat may be a minimal or major component (Figure 5-35).

The epithelial elements also are highly variable. There may be a predominance of ducts surrounded by fibrous tissue, creating a pattern similar to gynecomastia. In other lesions, lobules predominate, and these can be normal or atrophic. The ductules can be closely apposed or widely separated by stroma, thereby adding to the diversity of microscopic images.

Myoid Hamartoma

Daroca et al reported three cases of what they term *myoid hamartoma* of the breast. These lesions are distinctive, microscopically, from the hamartoma described above and consist of well-demarcated nodules of smooth muscle, sometimes intermixed with sclerosing adenosis, as well as fat. The described patients were 38, 39, and 61 years of age. Oberman also has described small foci of smooth muscle in hamartomas of the type described above.

Adenolipoma

Haagensen reported 43 adenolipomas occurring in women with a mean age of 44 years. Adenolipomas form palpable masses that are well circumscribed and may have been present for several years. They also may be identified on mammograms (Dyreborg and Starklint). Grossly, adenolipomas are indistinguishable from an ordinary soft tissue lipoma. Microscopically, varying numbers of small ducts and lobules are present within adipose tissue (Figure 5-36). Whether these are merely residual breast tissue infiltrated by fat (analogous to infiltrating lipomas in skeletal muscle) or a participating component of the proliferation is a moot point. The fact that the lobules often directly abut the fat and individual ductules are separated by adipose tissue suggests that infiltration is the better explanation. Lobular carcinoma in situ has been reported in one adenolipoma (Mendiola et al). Adenolipoma does not appear, however, to have any special predilection for the development of epithelial abnormalities.

Ordinary lipomas of the breast are far more common than adenolipomas. Mammary lipomas occur in all decades of life but are most common between the ages of 40 and 60 years. Haagensen described 292 such lesions.

REFERENCES

Adami HG, Hakaelius L, Rimsten A, et al. Malignant locally recurrent cystosarcoma in an adolescent female. *Acta Chir Scand* 1984;150: 93-100.

Ali M, Fayemi AO, Braun EV, Remy R. Fibromatosis of the breast. *Am J Surg Pathol* 1979; 3:501-505.

Amerson JR. Cystosarcoma phyllodes in adolescent females. A report of seven patients. *Ann Surg* 1970;171:849-858.

Arrigoni MG, Dockerty MB, Judd ES. The identification and treatment of mammary hamartoma. *Surg Gynecol Obstet* 1971;133;577-582.

Azzopardi JG. *Problems in Breast Pathology.* WB Saunders Co, Philadelphia, 1979, p 42.

Berean K, Tron VA, Churg A, Clement PB. Mammary fibroadenoma with multinucleated stromal giant cells. *Am J Surg Pathol* 1986; 10:823-827.

Case TC. Adenocarcinoma of breast. Arising in adenoma. *NY State J Med* 1977;77:2122-2123.

Daroca PJ Jr, Reed RJ, Love GL, Kraus SD. Myoid hamartomas of the breast. *Hum Pathol* 1985; 16:212-219.

Dêschenes L, Jacob S, Fabia J, Christen A. Beware of breast fibroadenomas in middle-aged women. *Can J Surg* 1985;28:372-374.

Diaz NM, Palmer JO, McDivitt RW. Carcinoma arising within a fibroadenoma of the breast. A clinicopathologic study of 105 patients. *Mod Pathol* 1990;3:26A.

DuPont WD, Page DL, Parl FF. Breast cancer risk associated with fibroadenomas. *Mod Pathol* 1990;3:28A.

Dyreborg U, Starklint H. Adenolipoma mammae. *Acta Radiol Diagn* 1975;16:362-366.

Fechner RE. Fibroadenomas in patients receiving oral contraceptives. A clinical and pathologic study. *Am J Clin Pathol* 1970;53:857-864.

Fekete P, Petrek J, Majmudar B, et al. Fibroadenomas with stromal cellularity. A clinicopathologic study of 21 patients. *Arch Pathol Lab Med* 1987;111:427-432.

Frantz VK, Pickren JW, Melcher GW, Auchinloss H Jr. Incidence of chronic cystic disease in so-called 'normal breasts.' A study based on 225 postmortem examinations. *Cancer* 1951; 4:762-783.

Grove A, Kristensen LD. Intraductal carcinoma within a phyllodes tumor of the breast. A case report. *Tumori* 1986;72:187-190.

Haagensen CD. *Diseases of the Breast*, ed 3. WB Saunders Co, Philadelphia, 1986, pp 290, 335-336.

Hart WR, Bauer RC, Oberman HA. Cytosarcoma phyllodes. A clinicopathological study of twenty-six hypercellular periductal stromal tumors of the breast. *Am J Clin Pathol* 1978; 70:211-216.

Hertel BF, Zaloudek C, Kempson RL. Breast adenomas. *Cancer* 1976;37:2891-2905.

Hessler C, Schnyder P, Ozzello L. Hamartoma of the breast. Diagnostic observation of 16 cases. *Radiology* 1978;126:995-998.

Hill RP, Miller FN Jr. Adenomas of the breast. With case report of carcinomatous transformation in an adenoma. *Cancer* 1954;7:318-324.

Hogeman KE, Östberg G. Three cases of postlactational breast tumor of a peculiar type. *Acta Pathol Microbiol Scand* 1968;73:169-176.

Huntrakoon M, Lin F. Muscular hamartoma of the breast. An electron microscopic study. *Virchows Arch Pathol Anat A* 1984;403:306-321.

Knudsen PJT, Østergaard J. Cystosarcoma phylloides with lobular and ductal carcinoma in situ. *Arch Pathol Lab Med* 1987;111:873-875.

Kodlin D, Winger EE, Morgenstern NL, Chen U. Chronic mastopathy and breast cancer. A follow-up study. *Cancer* 1977;39:2603-2607.

Kovi J, Chu HB, Leffall LD Jr. Sclerosing lobular hyperplasia manifesting as a palpable mass of the breast in young black women. *Hum Pathol* 1984;15:336-340.

LeGal Y. Adenomas of the breast. Relationship of adenofibroma to pregnancy and lactation. *Am Surg* 1961;27:14-22.

Linell F, Östberg G, Söderström J, et al. Breast hamartomas. An important entity in mammary pathology. *Virchows Arch A* 1979;383: 253-264.

LiVolsi VA, Stadel BV, Kelsey JL, Holford TR. Fibroadenoma in oral contraceptive users. A histopathologic evaluation of epithelial atypia. *Cancer* 1979;44:1778-1781.

Majmudar B, Rosales-Quintana S. Infarction of breast fibroadenomas during pregnancy. *JAMA* 1975;231:963-964.

Mendiola H, Henrik-Nielson R, Dyreborg U, et al. Lobular carcinoma in situ occurring in adenolipoma of the breast. Report of a case. *Acta Radiol Diagn* 1982;23:503-505.

Mies C, Rosen PP. Juvenile fibroadenoma with atypical epithelial hyperplasia. *Am J Surg Pathol* 1987;11:184-190.

Moross T, Lang AP, Mahoney L. Tubular adenoma of breast. *Arch Pathol Lab Med* 1983;107:84-86.

Morris JA, Kelley JF. Multiple bilateral breast adenomata in identical adolescent Negro twins. *Histopathology* 1982;6:539-547.

Moskowitz M, Gartside P, Wirman JA, McLaughlin C. Proliferative disorders of the breast as risk factors for breast cancer in a self-selected screened population. Pathologic markers. *Radiology* 1980;134:289-291.

Oberman HA. Breast lesions in the adolescent female. *Pathol Annu* 1979;14(part 1):175-201.

Oberman HA. Hamartomas and hamartoma variants of the breast. *Semin Diagn Pathol* 1989; 6:135-145.

O'Hara MF, Page DL. Adenomas of the breast and ectopic breast under lactational influences. *Hum Pathol* 1985;16:707-712.

Oliver RL, Major RC. Cyclomastopathy. A physiopathologic conception of some benign breast tumors with an analysis of four hundred cases. *Am J Cancer* 1934;21:1-85.

Ozzello L, Gump FE. The management of patients with carcinomas in fibroadenomatous tumors of the breast. *Surg Gynecol Obstet* 1985;160: 99-104.

Persaud V, Talerman A, Jordan RP. Pure adenoma of the breast. *Arch Pathol* 1968;86:481-483.

Petrik PK. Mammary hamartoma. *Am J Surg Pathol* 1987;11:234-235.

Pick PW, Iossifides IA: Occurrence of breast carcinoma within a fibroadenoma. A review. *Arch Pathol Lab Med* 1984;108:590-594.

Pike AM, Oberman HA. Juvenile (cellular) adenofibromas. A clinicopathologic study. *Am J Surg Pathol* 1985;9:730-736.

Rickert RR, Rajan S. Localized breast infarcts associated with pregnancy. *Arch Pathol* 1974; 97:159-162.

Ward RM, Evans HL. Cystosarcoma phyllodes. A clinicopathologic study of 26 cases. *Cancer* 1986;58:2282-2289.

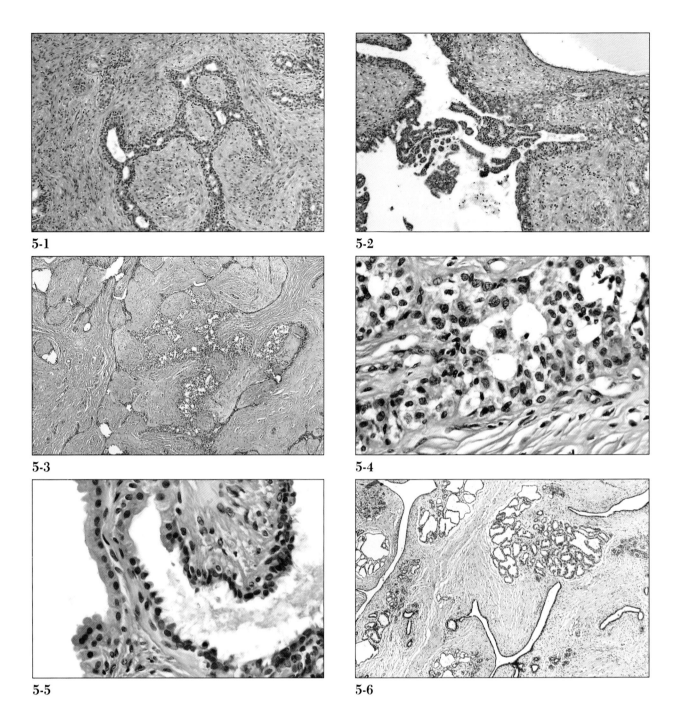

5-1

5-2

5-3

5-4

5-5

5-6

Figure 5-1. Anastomosing ductules with a visible myoepithelial cell layer are located in a fibroblastic stroma. Apparent bridging of ductular epithelium due to tangential sectioning is common and does not represent hyperplasia.

Figure 5-3. Often, epithelial proliferations in fibroadenoma may have a cribriform appearance at low magnification.

Figure 5-5. Apocrine metaplasia is present in approximately 14% of fibroadenomas.

Figure 5-2. Hyperplasia may be present in fibroadenoma and form irregular papillary structures. The epithelial cells are identical to those in nonhyperplastic foci and the cytologic features of micropapillary carcinoma are absent (pages 125 and 126).

Figure 5-4. Higher magnification of Figure 5-3 shows variable epithelial cells that are randomly oriented with respect to lumen-like spaces. These features are characteristic of hyperplasia (see page 92).

Figure 5-6. Lactational change may be seen in fibroadenomas during pregnancy and, as in this case, in women using oral contraceptives.

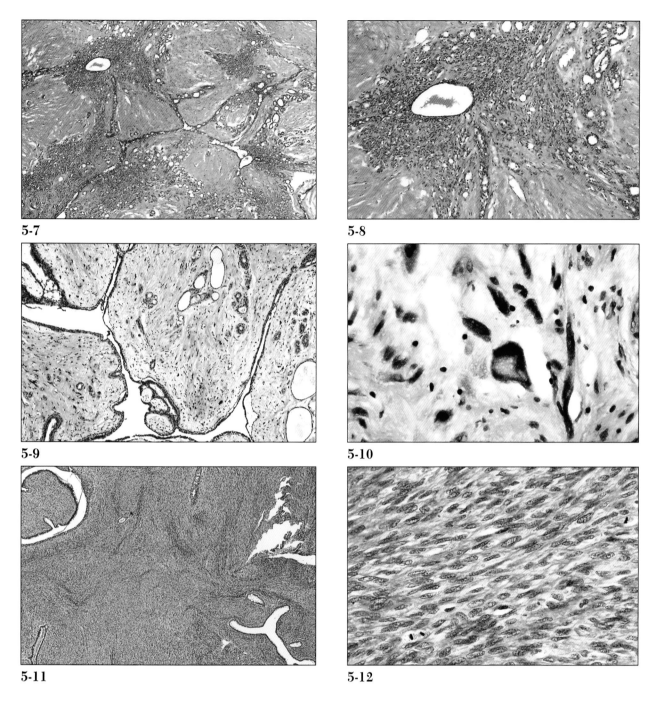

5-7

5-8

5-9

5-10

5-11

5-12

Figure 5-7. Sclerosing adenosis may be present in fibroadenoma, reflecting the lobular origin of the epithelial component.

Figure 5-9. Fibroadenomas may contain scattered atypical stromal cells with enlarged nuclei. Overall stromal cellularity is not increased, however.

Figure 5-11. Phyllodes tumor has stromal overgrowth manifested by widely separated glands.

Figure 5-8. At higher magnification, sclerosing adenosis in a fibroadenoma forms cords of cells with scattered lumina. The latter are often larger peripherally, as is typical of sclerosing adenoma (page 61).

Figure 5-10. At higher magnification, the atypical stromal cells of a fibroadenoma have densely hyperchromatic, angulated nuclei. A multinucleated stromal cell also is present.

Figure 5-12. The stroma of phyllodes tumor is cellular, but it lacks the giant cells sometimes seen in fibroadenomas.

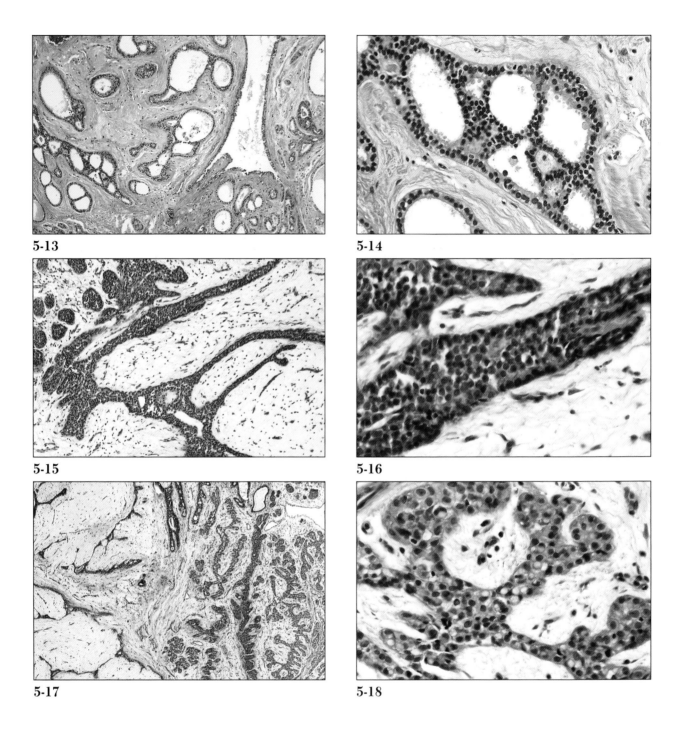

5-13

5-14

5-15

5-16

5-17

5-18

Figure 5-13. Micropapillary ductal carcinoma in situ (left) may arise in a fibroadenoma.

Figure 5-15. Lobular carcinoma in situ is the most common form of noninvasive carcinoma seen in fibroadenomas.

Figure 5-17. The junction of lobular carcinoma in situ (right) with uninvolved fibroadenoma (left) is clearly seen. Partial involvement of this type is common.

Figure 5-14. A higher magnification of Figure 5-13 demonstrates a monomorphic population of cells with typical architectural features of micropapillary carcinoma. This contrasts with the cellular variation seen in fibroadenoma-associated hyperplasia (Figures 5-2 to 5-4).

Figure 5-16. A higher magnification of Figure 5-15 demonstrates the monomorphic cell population of lobular carcinoma in situ (pages 155 through 158).

Figure 5-18. The lobular carcinoma in situ in this fibroadenoma demonstrates characteristic target cells (see page 150).

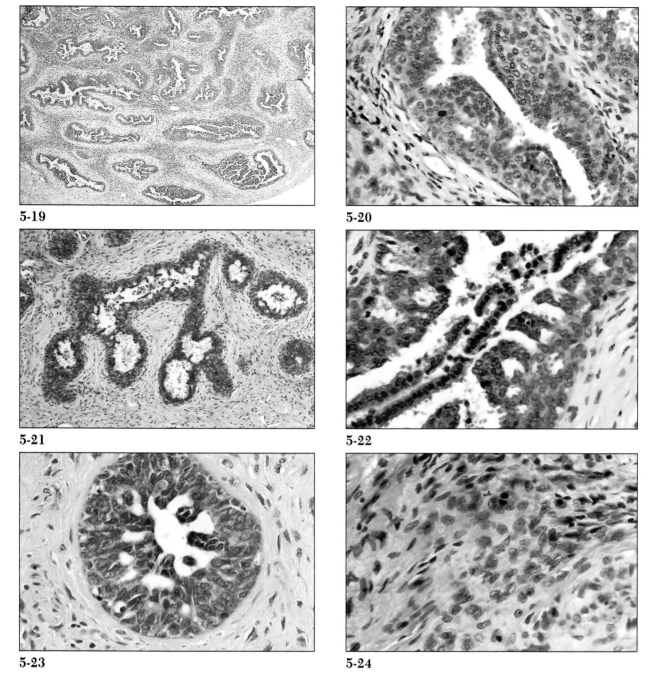

5-19

5-20

5-21

5-22

5-23

5-24

Figure 5-19. Juvenile fibroadenoma has more cellular stroma and more prominent epithelial hyperplasia than typical adult-type fibroadenoma. The low-power pattern, unlike adult-type fibroadenoma, resembles florid gynecomastia.

Figure 5-21. Lumina in juvenile fibroadenoma may occasionally contain exfoliated cellular debris. Epithelial bridges and small papillae are also present.

Figure 5-23. The tips of papillae in juvenile fibroadenoma often have smaller cells with denser nuclei. This is not a typical feature of micropapillary carcinoma. Mild nuclear atypia is present, however.

Figure 5-20. The epithelial hyperplasia in juvenile fibroadenoma consists of cells with variably shaped, often overlapping nuclei. In this field, the luminal layer of epithelial cells is focally flattened.

Figure 5-22. At higher magnification, the epithelium of juvenile fibroadenoma forms looping bridges and vertical papillae. Exfoliated strips of epithelium are also present in the lumen.

Figure 5-24. Stroma of juvenile fibroadenoma may be hypercellular, with considerable nuclear pleomorphism.

42

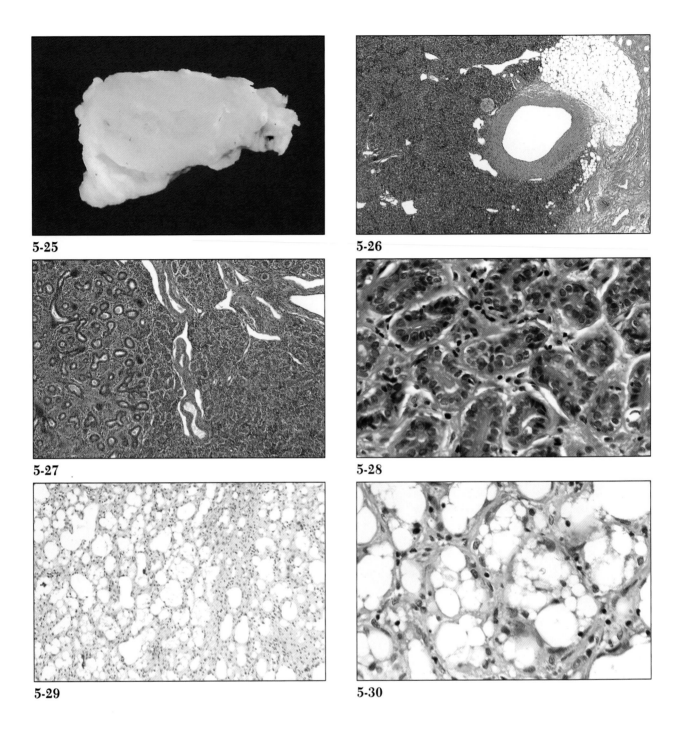

5-25

5-26

5-27

5-28

5-29

5-30

Figure 5-25. Tubular adenomas are sharply circumscribed and tan or yellow.

Figure 5-27. The ductules of tubular adenoma are individually indistinguishable from normal breast and show the same variation in diameter.

Figure 5-29. Lactating adenoma has the overall architecture of tubular adenoma but exhibits marked lactational change.

Figure 5-26. The margin of tubular adenoma is irregular. Nerves, vessels, and adipose tissue may be engulfed by the lesion.

Figure 5-28. In this tubular adenoma, the ductules contain secretions and myoepithelial cells are only occasionally visible.

Figure 5-30. The cells of lactating adenoma have copious amounts of vacuolated cytoplasm. These hormonally stimulated lesions often exhibit mild nuclear pleomorphism.

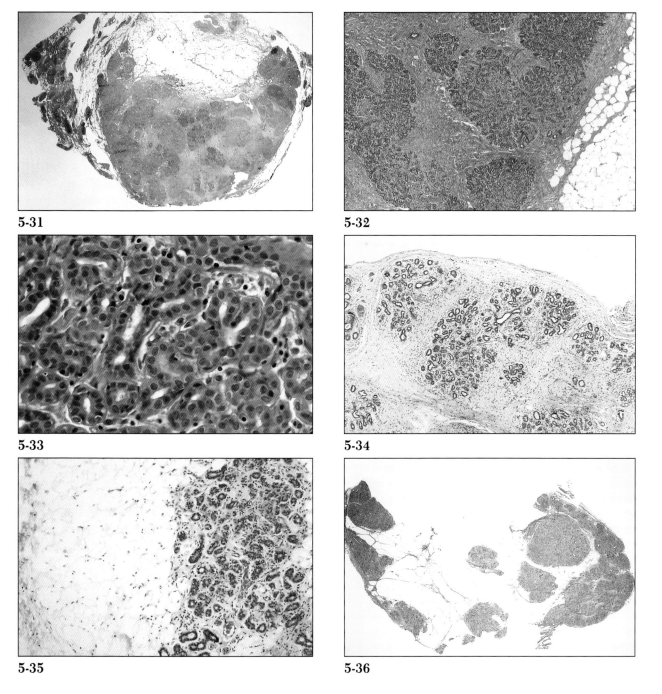

5-31

5-32

5-33

5-34

5-35

5-36

Figure 5-31. Sclerosing lobular hyperplasia usually forms a sharply circumscribed palpable mass.

Figure 5-33. The ductules of sclerosing lobular hyperplasia may be both closely packed and branching.

Figure 5-35. A higher magnification of Figure 5-34 shows juxtaposition of fat and irregularly scattered ductules typical of hamartoma.

Figure 5-32. Sclerosing lobular hyperplasia consists of confluent lobules and dense stroma.

Figure 5-34. Hamartomas are sharply circumscribed and consist of lobules of varying size intermixed with fibrous stroma and adipose tissue (Figure 5-35).

Figure 5-36. So-called adenolipoma is a sharply circumscribed mass composed of irregular aggregates of lobules interspersed in adipose tissue. During slide preparation, the central area of fat has been artifactually disrupted.

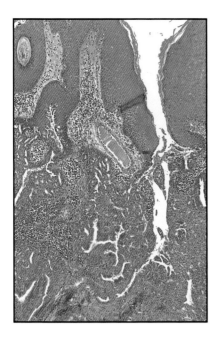

6

NIPPLE ADENOMA AND SUBAREOLAR PAPILLOMATOSIS

The benign epithelial proliferations that occur frequently in the region of the nipple have been the subject of numerous papers that have resulted in an almost equal number of diagnostic terms. We prefer to separate these lesions into those that clearly involve the nipple (nipple adenoma), and those that are located in the subareolar tissue but do not involve the nipple itself (subareolar papillomatosis). The proliferations in these two locations frequently have overlapping histologic appearances, but may differ in their clinical features.

NIPPLE ADENOMA

Lesions of the nipple that are characterized by complex proliferations of epithelium intermixed with varying amounts of fibrous tissue have been referred to as *papillary adenomas, nipple adenomas, adenomatosis,* and *erosive adenomatosis.* An additional term, *florid papillomatosis,* was used by Jones et al in 1955 in the first major publication dealing with benign tumors of the nipple. We prefer the term nipple adenoma because it is simple, accurate, and generic. Nipple adenomas are distinct from intraductal papillomas that occasionally arise within the lactiferous sinus and are located partly or completely within the nipple. The proliferating epithelium of

nipple adenomas is in continuity with the squamous epithelium of the nipple (Figure 6-1), although such continuity may not always be demonstrable because of variations in the plane of sectioning.

Nipple adenoma may occur at any age. Rosen and Caicco reported one lesion that was present at birth and another that was diagnosed at age 89. The majority of nipple adenomas, however, occur in patients between the ages of 35 and 65 years. The most common complaint is nipple discharge or crusting. Physical examination usually shows a slightly irregular surface of the nipple. Sometimes it is eroded or ulcerated, and occasionally there is an underlying palpable nodule. Nipple adenomas have been described in males, including one patient being treated with diethylstilbestrol.

Nipple adenomas rarely recur after excision. Only one of 51 patients described by Perzin and Lattes had a local recurrence, probably because of an inadequate initial resection. One patient in their study developed carcinoma of the same breast 17 years later, and two had carcinoma of the opposite breast. This frequency of carcinoma is within the range of expectations for a normal population, and nipple adenomas are not viewed as markers of increased risk for carcinoma.

The microscopic appearance of the nipple adenoma is extremely diverse. Rosen and

Caicco divided their patients into four groups that reflect this microscopic spectrum. The largest group had a sclerosing papillomatosis pattern resembling sclerosing adenosis, in which the epithelium predominantly formed small ductules distorted by prominent fibrous tissue (Figure 6-2). Some of the larger ductules had florid hyperplasia of the usual type, as described in the section on fibrocystic changes. About one third of the cases with hyperplasia had focal necrosis within the hyperplastic epithelium. Apocrine metaplasia was also occasionally seen. There was hyperplasia of the overlying squamous epithelium of the nipple, and squamous cysts were frequently formed near the superficial ends of the ducts as they opened onto the nipple surface.

The second group of nipple adenomas, called the papillomatosis pattern, included the youngest and oldest patients in their series. Microscopically, lesions in this group had a minimal fibrous component and consisted of complex epithelial proliferations involving ducts of various sizes located immediately beneath the nipple (Figures 6-3, 6-4). Mitotic figures and focal necrosis were seen within the same lesions and independently (Figure 6-5). Hyperplastic duct epithelium replaced part or all of the surface epithelium of the nipple in some instances.

The adenosis pattern of nipple adenoma consisted of small ducts about the size of normal ductules or terminal ducts. Lesions with this pattern tended to be circumscribed, although not encapsulated. Mitotic figures and necrosis were absent from the three adenomas in this group.

Finally, 17 of the nipple adenomas reported by Rosen and Caicco were composed of mixtures of the three microscopic patterns just described. This subdivision of nipple adenomas into three microscopically diverse "pure" patterns and a mixed pattern illustrates the marked variation that nipple adenomas can display.

SYRINGOMATOUS ADENOMA

Nipple adenoma should be distinguished from a distinctive, locally invasive lesion described by Rosen and Caicco as "syringomatous adenoma of the nipple," and later by Jones et al as "infiltrating syringomatous adenoma of the nipple." These lesions are microscopically identical to the so-called microcystic adnexal carcinoma or sclerosing sweat duct carcinoma of the skin described by Cooper et al, as well as by others. Convincing arguments can be made for not labeling the breast lesions as malignant, however, to avoid physician confusion and potential overtreatment. The two studies of the breast include 15 lesions seen in women from 11 to 67 years of age, and a single case in a 76-year-old man. Infiltrating syringomatous adenoma is characterized by a proliferation of duct-like structures that are lined by a layer two or three cells thick (Figure 6-6). The proliferating ducts are haphazardly arranged around the normal large ducts in the nipple. Small keratin cysts are commonly encountered. Jones et al noted that all 11 lesions in their study had infiltrative margins, ten invaded the smooth muscle of the nipple, four extended into the underlying breast tissue, and one showed perineural invasion.

One woman with infiltrating syringomatous adenoma in Rosen's study had persisting, enlarging lesions over a 22-year span after incomplete excision, but other lesions did not demonstrate an aggressive course. Jones et al noted a recurrence rate of 45% following local excision, but these were controlled by reexcision. Metastases from infiltrating syringomatous adenoma have not been described, although we have seen an example of this lesion involve an axillary lymph node by direct extension from the overlying skin.

In addition to distinguishing infiltrating syringomatous adenoma from nipple adenoma, the former lesion must also be distinguished from tubular carcinoma. Seven of 11 cases in the study by Jones et al had been suspected of being tubular carcinomas. Although infiltrating syringomatous adenoma may superficially involve the breast parenchyma, it is centered in the nipple and subareolar tissue. Tubular carcinomas commonly occur deeper in the breast, often in the upper outer quadrant. The branching, complex tubules of infiltrating syringomatous adenoma are in contrast with the simple tubules with wide lumina that characterize tubular carcinoma. More importantly, the tubules of infiltrating syringomatous adenoma have a two-cell, epithelial-myoepithelial layer, whereas most of those in tubular carcinoma have a single layer of epithelial cells.

SUBAREOLAR PAPILLOMATOSIS

Epithelial proliferations that are qualitatively similar to nipple adenomas may occur beneath the areola without involving the nipple (Figure 6-7). Such lesions have been referred to as *subareolar sclerosing duct hyperplasia* and *subareolar papillomatosis.* We prefer the term subareolar papillomatosis because not all examples have a prominent sclerotic component. Subareolar papillomatosis should be distinguished from intraductal papillomas that involve the large ducts just beneath the nipple.

Subareolar papillomatosis occurs in women between 25 and 75 years of age. Most are in their 30s and 40s. Patients may have nipple discharge in association with a palpable mass that ranges from 0.6 to 2 cm in diameter. Nipple retraction is rare. Complete excision is almost always curative, and local recurrence probably reflects incomplete removal of the original lesion. On gross examination, subareolar papillomatosis appears as a round or oval mass with indistinct margins. The color is typically gray or brown, and dense fibrous tissue, occasionally with yellow streaks, may surround the mass. Microscopically, a broad spectrum of changes can be seen (Figures 6-8 to 6-10). The proliferating ducts form complex, branching patterns and vary greatly in size, ranging from structures resembling terminal ducts to large ducts of the size normally seen near the nipple. Some of the larger ducts are probably preexistent structures, and these may contain proliferating epithelium that assumes two major configurations. In one pattern, the epithelial cells line fibrovascular cores, producing intraductal papillomas identical to those described on pages 68 and 69. Other ducts in subareolar papillomatosis may contain florid hyperplasia of the usual type (Figures 6-9, 6-10). There may be moderate nuclear atypia in such foci (Figure 6-8), and focal epithelial cell necrosis also may be seen (Figure 6-10). There also may be proliferating ductules and occasional ductular aggregates resembling lobules. The large ducts and ductules may be haphazardly intermixed, with one or the other predominating in a given high-power field.

Fibrous tissue is sometimes abundant in subareolar papillomatosis, especially centrally, creating an overall appearance similar to that of a radial scar (Figure 6-11). Dilated ducts without hyperplasia may be present at the periphery of subareolar papillomatosis, furthering the resemblance to radial scar. Indeed, some examples of subareolar papillomatosis probably represent superficially located radial scars; at least they are microscopically indistinguishable from such lesions. Ducts in areas of sclerosis often have a prominent peripheral myoepithelial cell layer (Figure 6-12).

Intraductal carcinoma was found in one of the 12 cases of subareolar papillomatosis reported by Rosen. Focal intraductal carcinoma was also found in the subsequent mastectomy specimen from this patient. At present, however, subareolar papillomatosis is not considered a risk factor for subsequent carcinoma.

REFERENCES

Cooper PH, Mills SE, Leonard DD, et al. Sclerosing sweat duct (syringomatous) carcinoma. *Am J Surg Pathol* 1985;9:422-433.

Jones DB. Florid papillomatosis of the nipple ducts. *Cancer* 1955;8:315-319.

Jones MW, Norris HJ, Snyder RC. Infiltrating syringomatous adenoma of the nipple. A clinical and pathological study of 11 cases. *Am J Surg Pathol* 1989;13:197-201.

Perzin KH, Lattes R. Papillary adenoma of the nipple (florid papillomatosis, adenoma, adenomatosis). A clinicopathologic study. *Cancer* 1972;29:996-1009.

Rosen PP. Subareolar sclerosing duct hyperplasia of the breast. *Cancer* 1987;59:1927-1930.

Rosen PP. Syringomatous adenoma of the nipple. *Am J Surg Pathol* 1983;7:739-745.

Rosen PP, Caicco JA. Florid papillomatosis of the nipple. A study of 51 patients, including nine with mammary carcinoma. *Am J Surg Pathol* 1986;10:87-101.

Waldo ED, Sidhu GS, Hu AW. Florid papillomatosis of male nipple after diethylstilbestrol therapy. *Arch Pathol* 1975;99:364-366.

Ward BE, Cooper PH, Subramony C. Syringomatous tumor of the nipple. *Am J Clin Pathol* 1989;92:692-696.

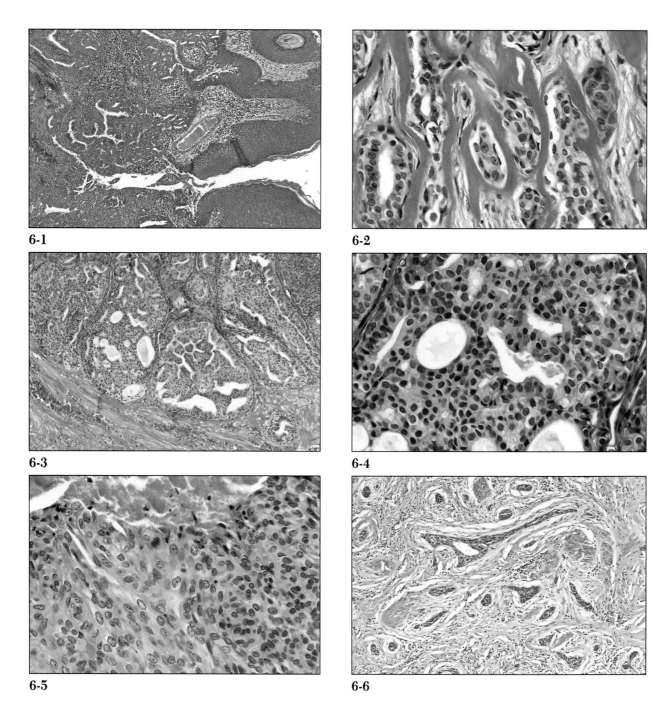

6-1

6-2

6-3

6-4

6-5

6-6

Figure 6-1. The proliferating ductal epithelium of nipple adenoma is contiguous with the squamous epithelium of the nipple surface.

Figure 6-3. Nipple adenomas may form duct-like structures with complex papillary architecture or irregular lumina.

Figure 6-5. Necrosis may be seen occasionally in nipple adenoma. Note that the cells have the cytologic features of hyperplasia as seen in Figure 6-4.

Figure 6-2. The proliferating epithelium of nipple adenoma may form sharply circumscribed nests separated by dense collagen. Lumina may or may not be visible.

Figure 6-4. The epithelium of nipple adenoma displays the cytologic variation typical of usual hyperplasia (see page 92).

Figure 6-6. Infiltrating syringomatous adenoma near the nipple extends between smooth muscle bundles. The irregular, sharply angulated cell nests have "comma-like" tails and occasional lumina.

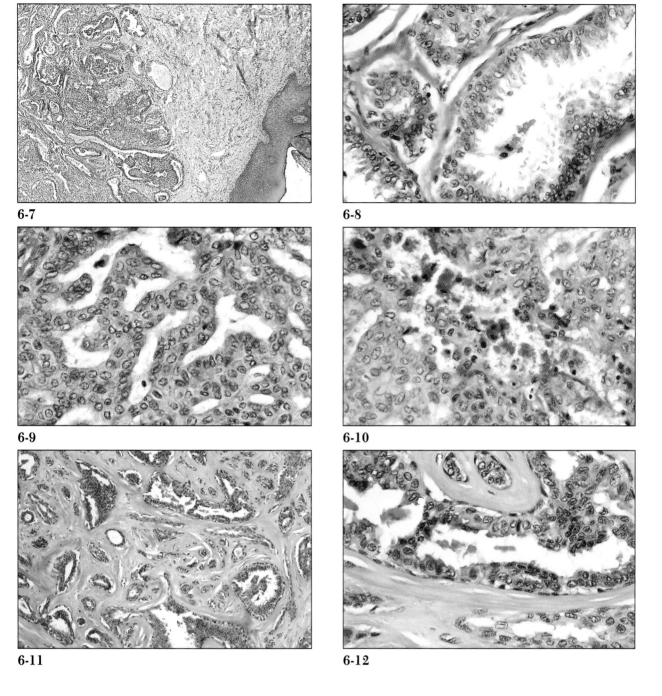

6-7

6-8

6-9

6-10

6-11

6-12

Figure 6-7. Subareolar papillomatosis occurs beneath the nipple without involving the overlying skin.

Figure 6-9. Serpiginous strands of epithelium in subareolar papillomatosis outline irregular spaces. The nuclei are imperfectly oriented with respect to the spaces.

Figure 6-11. Marked desmoplasia, usually located centrally, may be a component of subareolar papillomatosis. Such foci are indistinguishable from radial scars (page 52).

Figure 6-8. Although the epithelium is stratified and seemingly disorganized, it has the features of hyperplasia.

Figure 6-10. Necrosis may be seen in subareolar papillomatosis. The adjacent cells are identical to those previously illustrated.

Figure 6-12. Flattened but clearly visible myoepithelial cells are present beneath irregular, hyperplastic epithelium.

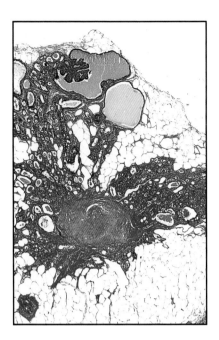

7

RADIAL SCAR, SCLEROSING ADENOSIS, AND ADENOSIS TUMOR

Many benign, microscopically compact epithelial proliferations originating in the lobule have varying degrees of stromal-associated proliferation. The stromal component may be fibrous, elastotic, or both. The interplay of the epithelial and stromal elements within the lobule results in a variety of reproducible microscopic images. Based on their low-power features, these proliferations are typically separated into such diagnostic categories as *radial scar*, *sclerosing adenosis*, and *adenosis tumor*. This chapter reviews the microscopic features of these benign, although microscopically complex, proliferations that may cause considerable diagnostic confusion with infiltrating carcinoma.

RADIAL SCAR

Radial scars have been recognized for more than 50 years and are referred to by a variety of terms, including *sclerosing papillary proliferation*, *nonencapsulated sclerosing lesion*, *infiltrating epitheliosis*, *indurative mastopathy*, and *benign sclerosing ductal proliferation*. These differing names highlight varying components of the lesion that are conspicuous in some cases and less obvious or absent in others. For example, *sclerosing papillary proliferation* emphasizes the epithelial hyperplasia of radial scar that may occasionally have a papillary architecture. *Nonencapsulated sclerosing lesion* emphasizes the lack of marginal fibrosis, and the term *infiltrating epitheliosis* distinguishes radial scar from intraductal epithelial proliferations. *Indurative mastopathy* emphasizes a radiographically detectable lesion that usually has fibrous tissue as the major component. Carter does not regard indurative mastopathy as synonymous with radial scar (Andersen et al, 1986). Page and Anderson limit the term radial scar to lesions up to 1 centimeter in diameter, and they use the phrase "complex sclerosing lesions" for larger proliferations having similar qualitative features. These different preferences for terminology reflect an uncertainty regarding the homogeneity of the mixed epithelial and fibrous proliferations denoted by the term *radial scar*. Indeed, radial scars may have different pathogeneses. Carter has presented several hypothetical pathways by which the final image of a radial scar might be attained (Andersen et al, 1986). Nevertheless, examination of published photographs to which the above terms have been applied shows at least some overlap of the images, and it is expeditious for the purposes of this discussion to encompass them with a single term. At present, the term *radial scar* enjoys popularity and has the virtue of brevity.

Radial scars are common. Fisher et al found them in 15 (4%) of 400 consecutive biopsy specimens obtained for fibrocystic changes and in 4% of random sections from mastectomy specimens removed for carcinoma. Wellings and Alpers, using the subgross method of examination, studied 83 breasts at autopsy from women without a history of mammary carcinoma and found that 14% contained one to 13 radial scars. In the same series, 26% of breasts from patients with prior mammary carcinoma had radial scars. The average number of radial scars per breast was higher in the latter group, ranging from one to 31. However, Nielsen et al (1985) found no difference in the frequency of radial scars in women with a history of breast cancer, as compared with women having either normal breasts or breasts containing benign abnormalities.

In routinely examined tissue sections, the frequency of radial scars is undoubtedly underestimated. Serial section studies, including our own, indicate that many foci of apparent sclerosing adenosis or intraductal hyperplasia are actually the edges of radial scars in sections that do not cut through the central fibrotic zone.

Follow-up of patients who had radial scars in benign biopsy specimens is available in one study. Andersen and Gram found radial scars in 84 patients who were followed up for at least 15 years. One woman developed carcinoma, but the risk was calculated to be the same as for the general population. Because radial scars are often associated with a variety of epithelial proliferations, multivariant analysis would be required to evaluate them as an independent risk factor for carcinoma. Such information is currently unavailable, however. Carcinoma arising in radial scars is discussed below.

A small proportion of radial scars is palpable or visualized mammographically. Rarely, they are fixed to skin or associated with nipple discharge (Fenoglio and Lattes, Rickert et al). In gross specimens, radial scars range from 0.5 to 1.3 cm in size, and can be as firm to palpation as the usual infiltrating ductal or lobular carcinoma. A stellate pattern of gray or yellow streaks is typical (Figure 7-1). A few small cysts may be identifiable at the edge of the lesion. These macroscopic radial scars are impossible to distinguish from infiltrating carcinoma on gross examination.

Microscopically, radial scars are an epithelial proliferation that extends in a spoked wheel pattern from a central fibrotic area. Presumably, the earliest stage in the formation of a radial scar is a central area that is cellular with minimal collagen (Figures 7-2 to 7-4). Ultrastructurally, the cells have been shown to be myofibroblasts associated with atrophic ductules (Battersby and Anderson). Later stages of radial scar are manifested by a sparsely cellular, densely collagenized center that may have many elastic fibers (Figures 7-5, 7-6). In fact, Wellings and Alpers require that the central portions have fibroelastotic tissue before using the term radial scar. The amount of epithelium in the fibrous areas varies in an approximately inverse relationship to the density of the connective tissue. The denser, fibrotic foci have haphazardly distributed nests, cords, or individual epithelial cells. At high power, the random arrangement of these cells is indistinguishable from the pattern of an infiltrating carcinoma (Figures 7-7, 7-8). As alluded to above, the epithelial proliferation peripheral to the central fibroelastotic zone has components that are indistinguishable from sclerosing adenosis and hyperplasia of the usual type (Figures 7-9 to 7-12). The same microscopic criteria discussed in the sections on sclerosing adenosis (page 53) and ductal hyperplasia (page 92) are applied to the epithelial components of radial scar to distinguish these elements from carcinoma.

At the edges of a radial scar, there are often normal-sized to widely dilated ductules (Figure 7-5). Some of the larger peripheral lumina are probably terminal ducts, either within or adjacent to lobules. The ductules or terminal ducts may be lined by a single or double layer of epithelium, or they may be hyperplastic. Lobules at the periphery of radial scars appear to be incorporated into radial scars by growth of the radiating fibroelastotic tissue. This would account for the preservation of well-formed lumina at the periphery of many lesions before their distortion by the scar.

Differential Diagnosis/Associated Lesions

The central elastotic area of radial scar mimics the elastotic, sparsely cellular foci of many infiltrating carcinomas (Figures 7-7, 7-8). Although a high-power field can have a growth pattern indistinguishable from that of carcinoma, examination of the lesion at medium or low power documents the architecture of a radial scar. In this setting, the disorganized epithelium in the central elastotic portion can be discounted as evidence of invasion.

Tubules lined by a single layer of cuboidal epithelium indistinguishable from tubular carcinoma are occasionally seen in radial scars, usually in the central or mid-portion of the scar. Only if there are multiple clear-cut myoepithelial cells can one be reasonably assured that a given ductule is not tubular carcinoma. Occasional cells thought to be myoepithelial cells have been seen in lesions interpreted as being tubular carcinoma (Erlandson and Carstens, Fisher et al).

It is our practice not to interpret ductules with a single layer of epithelium as being tubular carcinoma unless they are at the periphery of the radial scar and are unequivocally infiltrating the fat—an extremely rare finding. There is no magic number of tubules that must be present, but we suggest that at least a dozen are necessary in order to reasonably support the diagnosis of tubular carcinoma. From a practical standpoint, however, the presence of a few tubules that are indistinguishable from tubular carcinoma can be ignored. Carter has aptly summarized this situation by stating: "I would suggest that caution be exercised in the recognition of the tiniest tubular carcinoma for clinical purposes" (Andersen et al, 1986). Tubular carcinomas rarely metastasize to regional lymph nodes, and virtually all lesions that have done so have been 1 to 2 cm in size. Only one tubular carcinoma metastasized from a group of 101 carcinomas less than 1 cm in size (McDivitt et al). It is interesting that Anderson and Battersby in their detailed study of radial scars noted that tubular carcinomas bore a morphologic similarity to radial scars. Nevertheless, they were unable to establish criteria even in the "earliest" of invasive tubular cancers to support the concept that these carcinomas arose in radial scars.

Lobular and ductal carcinoma in situ are almost never seen in radial scars. Wellings and Alpers found no carcinomas in 92 radial scars from the breasts of women without a history of breast cancer. They also examined 434 radial scars associated with carcinoma in the ipsilateral or contralateral breast. Only a single radial scar contained ductal carcinoma in situ. Nielsen et al (1987) identified three women with invasive mammary carcinomas who had in their contralateral breasts a total of six radial scars containing in situ carcinomas. The carcinomas were equally divided between ductal and lobular carcinoma in situ subtypes.

In the event that lobular or ductal carcinoma in situ is found in a radial scar, it seems reasonable that the management of these patients be dictated by the features of their in situ carcinomas. Whether or not there is any biologic difference between carcinoma in situ arising in a radial scar as compared with other sites of origin is unknown.

SCLEROSING ADENOSIS

Sclerosing adenosis is a proliferation of lobular ductules and stroma (Figures 7-13 to 7-22). The clinical relevance of sclerosing adenosis as an independent risk factor for subsequent invasive carcinoma of the breast has been hinted at in the past (Kodlin et al). Recently, Jensen et al concluded that sclerosing adenosis was an independent risk factor that placed a woman at 1.7 times the risk of the general population. This is in the range of risk for lesions termed "proliferative breast disease without atypia." The study by Jensen et al is of further interest in that atypical lobular hyperplasia was present 2.7 times more frequently in breasts having sclerosing adenosis, as compared with breasts with fibrocystic changes and lacking this lesion. Sclerosing adenosis was not associated with atypical ductal hyperplasia. Cases with atypical lobular hyperplasia were not included in the calculations that led to the 1.7-fold increase in risk.

Sclerosing adenosis has an endless array of microscopic variations. The stroma can be cellular with many fibroblasts, or hypocellular and densely collagenized. Sclerosing adenosis is clearly of lobular origin, although, occasionally, areas indistinguishable from sclerosing adenosis are seen in solitary papillomas of large ducts. The ductules may retain well-formed lumina and have a double cell layer with an easily seen outer myoepithelial component. More often, however, no double layer is recognizable. The peripheral ductules of sclerosing adenosis tend to be of greater diameter than the central ones (Figure 7-13). In some examples of sclerosing adenosis, the epithelial cells exhibit minimal or absent lumen formation (Figures 7-14, 7-15). In these cases, the cells form cords from one to more than five cells thick. Nuclei range from round or ovoid to spindle-shaped; they may be small and densely staining or large and vesicular (Figure 7-16). In extremely cellular areas, the individual lobules of origin are no longer recognizable (Figure 7-17). The cells are often so closely packed that it is impossible to discern epithelial from myoepithelial cells (Figure 7-18). Microcalcifications are sometimes

54 prominent, but do not alter the overall appearance of the lesion (Figure 7-19). Apocrine metaplasia is an uncommon occurrence in sclerosing adenosis (Figure 7-20).

The proliferative epithelium of sclerosing adenosis can infiltrate the perineural space and this perineural "invasion" may also lead to confusion with carcinoma (Figure 7-23). Perineural involvement has been reported in approximately 2% of patients with sclerosing adenosis. Occasionally, epithelium may appear to be intraneural, an image probably produced by a tangential section through the involved perineural region (Figure 7-24). Vascular invasion has also been described as a rare finding in sclerosing adenosis (Eusebi and Azzopardi).

Differential Diagnosis

Isolated, atrophic lobules with collapsed lumina and increased interductular connective tissue somewhat resemble sclerosing adenosis but should not be diagnosed as such. Jensen et al require a focus of sclerosing adenosis to be at least double the size of adjacent, uninvolved lobules.

Larger examples of sclerosing adenosis removed because they produced a palpable mass, calcifications, or other mammographic abnormality are not as firm on gross examination as invasive carcinoma because of their lack of elastosis. Microscopically, foci of sclerosing adenosis lacking cytologic atypia are easily distinguished from infiltrating carcinoma. Although the disorderly cellular cords of sclerosing adenosis may be indistinguishable from infiltrating carcinoma under high-power magnification, the cytologic appearance is different. Perhaps the most helpful feature in separating sclerosing adenosis from infiltrating carcinoma is the low-power pattern. The periphery of sclerosing adenosis often has ductules that are rounded or "turned back," as if the peripheral ductules were being pushed in front of the lesion. This is in contrast to an irregular, infiltrating or dispersed cell pattern at the periphery of carcinoma. As mentioned above, sclerosing adenosis often has ductules that are larger at the periphery and small or absent centrally. Carcinoma lacks this feature.

Some lesions of sclerosing adenosis consist mainly of collagen with few epithelial or myoepithelial cells. These may represent foci of sclerosing adenosis that have become atrophic. Such foci must not be mistaken for infiltrating carcinoma. The scattered epithelial and myoepithelial cells in the dense stroma are cytologically benign and many have ovoid nuclei (Figures 7-21, 7-22). Cytoplasm is scant. Infiltrating lobular carcinoma is most likely to be confused with this image because it is composed of small cells. The cells of infiltrating lobular carcinoma, however, have slightly larger, uniform, round nuclei and more cytoplasm as compared with the atrophic cells in sclerosing adenosis.

Most diagnostic problems associated with sclerosing adenosis result from the occasional presence of severely atypical cells in this architectural setting. Large atypical cells cytologically indistinguishable from infiltrating ductal carcinoma may be present in sclerosing adenosis. Even in these situations, however, the low-power pattern of sclerosing adenosis is preserved, and this helpful feature should allow the distinction of carcinoma in situ in sclerosing adenosis from infiltrating carcinoma. The majority of cells in such foci will have bland nuclei, some of which will be ovoid or spindle-shaped, in contrast to infiltrating carcinoma. When benign epithelial cells of sclerosing adenosis are interspersed with the cords and nests of neoplastic cells, this combination can be used to distinguish noninvasive neoplasia in sclerosing adenosis from invasive carcinoma. In addition, the presence of large ductules at the periphery of the lesion, as is commonly seen in typical sclerosing adenosis, also aids in the distinction from invasive carcinoma. A greater diagnostic problem occurs when neoplastic cells form individual cords or small nests within sclerosing adenosis. Lobular carcinoma in situ also may involve foci of sclerosing adenosis. This is illustrated in the chapter dealing with lobular carcinoma in situ (page 150).

ADENOSIS TUMOR

Haagensen proposed the term *adenosis tumor* for confluent and intermingling lobules of sclerosing adenosis that produce a palpable mass. Other terms used for this condition include *palpable form of sclerosing adenosis, aggregate adenosis,* and *fibrosing adenomatosis.*

Adenosis tumor is usually solitary, but rarely may be multiple, and occasionally is bilateral. Most affected women are between 20 and 50 years of age, with a peak incidence in the fourth decade of life. On physical examination, the palpable mass may be tender, and can be partially fixed in the breast parenchyma. Rarely does the degree of fixation mimic that of a carcinoma, however. Adenosis tumor apparently regresses after menopause. Haagensen reported that one patient who underwent biopsy for a palpable adenosis tumor did not have the lesion excised completely, and it disappeared after menopause with no evidence of recurrence 11 years later.

In the study by Nielsen, five of 27 patients with adenosis tumor had an associated carcinoma, but he attributed this to selection factors. In contrast, although Haagensen found that five of 52 patients with adenosis tumor subsequently developed carcinoma, he concluded that this was a statistically significant increase in risk (relative risk of 5.2). He emphasized, however, that this increased risk applied only to patients with adenosis tumors and not microscopic forms of sclerosing adenosis. The carcinomas developed in the opposite breast in three of the five patients. Data on other potentially associated risk factors such as atypical epithelial hyperplasia were not given.

Grossly, adenosis tumors range from approximately 6 to 25 mm in diameter and have a highly variable appearance. They are gray or have brown areas representing zones of epithelial proliferation. The cut surface may be granular, and small cysts less than 3 mm in diameter are frequent. Rarely, chalky streaks of stromal elastosis are visible and may lead to confusion with carcinoma. Stromal elastosis is found in up to two thirds of the cases (Nielsen). Adenosis tumor is often sharply demarcated; a finding verified on microscopic examination (Figure 7-25).

A variety of different microscopic growth patterns has been illustrated. This diversity is reflected in the terms used to describe the microscopic appearance of adenosis tumors, including nodular sclerosing adenosis (Figure 7-25), classic sclerosing adenosis (Figure 7-26), tubular adenosis (Figures 7-27, 7-28), diffuse glandular pattern, blunt duct adenosis, periductal adenosis, and a pseudoinfiltrative pattern (Figures 7-29, 7-30).

Some adenosis tumors have not only architectural variation (Figures 7-31, 7-32) but a broad cytologic spectrum as well. This can include mucus-secreting cells (Figures 7-33, 7-34), cells with small nuclei and scant clear cytoplasm (Figure 7-35), and apocrine epithelium (Figure 7-36). If there are cysts in adenosis tumor, they are almost always lined by apocrine epithelium. The heterogeneity of these cell populations is helpful in recognizing the mass of proliferating epithelium as a

benign process. It is possible that some lesions interpreted as adenosis tumors are radial scars in which the central portion of the scar does not appear in the plane of section.

MICROGLANDULAR ADENOSIS

Microglandular adenosis is a microscopically distinctive, disorderly proliferation of ductules that may easily be confused with carcinoma. It may form a palpable mass or be an incidental finding in breast tissue removed for other reasons. Microglandular adenosis can often be detected by mammography, but it does not have a distinctive appearance. Women with this lesion have ranged in age from 28 to 82 years, but most are between 45 and 60 years of age. Palpable lesions have been present for as little as 1 week to as long as 5 years.

Grossly, microglandular adenosis has a variable, nonspecific appearance, much of which is attributable to the frequently intermixed fibrocystic changes. The area specifically affected by microglandular adenosis is not sharply circumscribed or encapsulated. It consists of nondescript fibrofatty tissue with variable firmness due to differing proportions of fibrous and adipose tissue.

Microscopically, the area involved by microglandular adenosis may be much larger than is suspected on gross examination. Tavassoli and Norris estimated that some lesions are up to 20 cm in size, based on microscopic study of multiple sections. Most lesions are 1 to 5 cm in greatest dimension, however. Microglandular adenosis is an infiltrative, haphazard proliferation of small, gland-like structures about the size of normal ductules. Three-dimensional reconstructions have not been performed, and it is unclear whether the gland-like structures are truly spherical or tubular in configuration. The fact that almost all such structures in a given plane of section are circular strongly favors the theory that they are spherical. Some of the gland-like structures do have small branches or elongations, but, for the sake of brevity, we will refer to them as glands.

The glands of microglandular adenosis are either interspersed in the stroma around and between normal ducts and lobules (Figure 7-37) or scattered in fat and fibrous tissue at a considerable distance from any breast parenchyma (Figure 7-38). The round to slightly oval glands are lined by a single layer of cuboidal epithelial cells that lack apical snouts. The cytoplasm may be clear or eosinophilic, and is occasionally granular. The lumina are usually well formed and often contain densely eosinophilic material that stains for mucicarmine, but the cytoplasm is mucicarmine-negative (Figure 7-39). Nuclei are round and uniform. Occasionally, the cytoplasm is more voluminous, resulting in smaller lumina (Figure 7-40). Ultrastructurally, the single layer of epithelial cells seen light microscopically directly abuts the stroma, and an intervening myoepithelial cell layer is absent. The cytoplasm may contain a few secretory droplets, but lacks distinctive features.

Both epithelial atypia and overt carcinoma have been described in association with microglandular adenosis. The atypical features occur at the histologic as well as the cytologic level. Histologic atypia is manifest by an increase in elongated glands, interconnecting glands, and glandular lumina of more variable size. Foci of atypical microglandular adenosis often have minimal or absent luminal secretory material. This more complex architectural appearance is usually accompanied by cytologically atypical cells characterized by larger, more pleomorphic, stratified nuclei with easily identifiable nucleoli (Figures 7-41, 7-42). The fate of atypical microglandular adenosis treated only by biopsy is unknown.

Microglandular adenosis is occasionally seen in breasts removed for ordinary infiltrating ductal carcinoma. In such instances, the adenosis is distant from the carcinoma, there is neither cytologic nor architectural overlap, and the lesions appear to be unrelated (Tavassoli and Norris). However, Rosenblum et al have demonstrated the close association of typical microglandular adenosis, atypical microglandular adenosis, and large rounded aggregates of atypical cells that appear to represent invasive carcinoma. The carcinomatous areas were intermixed with more irregularly shaped nests of cells, further supporting the diagnosis of invasive cancer. The apparent microscopic continuum from typical microglandular adenosis to carcinoma led Rosenblum et al to conclude that this lesion could give rise to malignancy. Although the carcinomatous components contained varying numbers of clear cells, the authors emphasized that eosinophilic cells with conspicuous cytoplasmic granularity should arouse suspicion of malignancy. Their eight patients with associated carcinoma account for 25% of the cases of microglandular adenosis that they have studied. Although experience with this unusual setting for carcinoma is limited, Rosenblum et al suggest that therapy should be the same as for other carcinomas at the same clinical stage.

One case reported by Rosenblum et al as intraductal carcinoma in microglandular adenosis was also reported by Kiaer et al, who interpreted the lesion as a low-grade malignant adenomyoepithelioma rather than intraductal carcinoma. Myoepithelial cells were identified by electron microscopy, as well as by immunohistochemical staining for actin. Such diverse interpretations of a single lesion by highly experienced pathologists serve as a reminder of the difficulty in classifying some of these rare, complex proliferations of the breast.

Differential Diagnosis

The differential diagnosis of microglandular adenosis includes sclerosing adenosis, adenomyoepithelial adenosis, and tubular carcinoma. Sclerosing adenosis, unlike microglandular adenosis, is oriented around the lobules from which it arises. Myoepithelial cells are often clearly visible, and a proliferating stromal component is common. These features usually allow ready distinction from microglandular adenosis. Nonetheless, the peripheral portions of sclerosing adenosis may contain more dispersed, small glands, and, in this region, there may be some overlap in microscopic appearances.

Adenomyoepithelial adenosis is a term that has been applied to gland-like structures composed of a double layer of epithelium. As the name implies, the outer layer consists of myoepithelial cells (Kiaer et al). As discussed under the section on adenomyoepithelioma (page 70), adenomyoepithelial adenosis appears to carry a definite risk of recurrence, in contrast to microglandular adenosis.

The distinction of microglandular adenosis from tubular carcinoma is extremely important. Grossly, most tubular carcinomas have a stellate configuration and are very firm, because of the associated elastosis. This differs from the nondescript, fibrocystic-like appearance of microglandular adenosis. Microscopically, tubular carcinoma not only has foci of elastic tissue but, usually, a marked desmoplastic response (Figures 7-43, 7-44). The most helpful distinguishing features are the cytologic and architectural differences in the glands. As discussed above, microglandular adenosis is predominantly composed of round glands, whereas tubular carcinomas contain a

56

much larger proportion of irregularly shaped, elongated glands (tubules). The glands or tubules of tubular carcinoma often appear to grow into and "split" the surrounding stroma. The periphery of a tubular carcinoma most closely resembles microglandular adenosis. The desmoplastic response seen in the central portion of a tubular carcinoma has not yet developed, and, therefore, the tubules have only a loose fibrous reaction or may lie within fat (Figures 7-45, 7-46). In these foci, one must rely on cytologic criteria. The cells of tubular carcinoma consistently have eosinophilic cytoplasm and often have apical "snouts." By contrast, most examples of microglandular adenosis contain clear cells, and apical snouts are invariably absent. Secretory material is rarely seen in the glandular lumina of tubular carcinoma, in contrast to microglandular adenosis. Some infiltrating ductal carcinomas have well-formed lumina such as are seen in tubular carcinoma. Their cytologic atypia, however, is far greater, allowing ready distinction from tubular carcinoma. These tubule-forming infiltrating carcinomas also can be distinguished from microglandular adenosis on the basis of their prominent cytologic abnormalities (Figures 7-47, 7-48).

REFERENCES

Anderson TJ, Battersby S. Radial scars of benign and malignant breasts. Comparative features and significance. *J Pathol* 1985;147:23-32.

Andersen JA, Carter D, Linell F. A symposium on sclerosing duct lesions of the breast. *Pathol Annu* 1986;21(part 2):145-179.

Andersen JA, Gram JB. Radial scar in the female breast. A long-term follow-up study of 32 cases. *Cancer* 1984;53:2557-2560.

Azzopardi JG. *Problems in Breast Pathology*. WB Saunders Co, Philadelphia, 1979, pp 174-188.

Battersby S, Anderson TJ. Myofibroblast activity of radial scars. *J Pathol* 1985;147:33-40.

Carter D, Rosen PP. Atypical sclerosing lesions. A study of 51 patients. *Mod Pathol* 1990;3:28A.

Clement PB, Azzopardi JG. Microglandular adenosis of the breast. A lesion simulating tubular carcinoma. *Histopathology* 1983;7:169-180.

Davies JD. Hyperelastosis, obliteration and fibrous plaques in major ducts of the human breast. *J Pathol* 1973;110:13-26.

Erlandson RA, Carstens PHB. Ultrastructure of tubular carcinoma of the breast. *Cancer* 1972;29:987-995.

Eusebi V, Azzopardi JG. Vascular infiltration in benign breast disease. *J Pathol* 1976;118:9-16.

Fechner RE. Lobular carcinoma *in situ* in sclerosing adenosis. A potential source of confusion with invasive carcinoma. *Am J Surg Pathol* 1981;5:233-239.

Fenoglio C, Lattes R. Sclerosing papillary proliferations in the female breast. A benign lesion often mistaken for carcinoma. *Cancer* 1974;33:691-700.

Fisher ER, Palekar AS, Kotwal N, Lipana N. A non-encapsulated sclerosing lesion of the breast. *Am J Clin Pathol* 1979;71:240-246.

Gould VE, Rogers DR, Sommers SC. Epithelial-nerve intermingling in benign breast lesions. *Arch Pathol* 1975;99:596-598.

Haagensen CD. *Diseases of the Breast*, ed 3. WB Saunders Co, Philadelphia, 1986, pp 106-117.

Jensen RA, Page DL, Dupont WD, Rogers LW. Invasive breast cancer risk in women with sclerosing adenosis. *Cancer* 1989;64:1977-1983.

Kay S. Microglandular adenosis of the female mammary gland. Study of a case with ultrastructural observations. *Hum Pathol* 1985;16:637-640.

Kiaer H, Nielsen B, Paulsen S, et al. Adenomyoepithelial adenosis and low-grade malignant adenomyoepithelioma of the breast. *Virchows Arch A* 1984;405:55-67.

Kodlin D, Winger EE, Morgenstern NL, Chen U. Chronic mastopathy and breast cancer. A follow-up study. *Cancer* 1977;39:2603-2607.

Linell F, Ljungberg O. Breast carcinoma. Progression of tubular carcinoma and a new classification. *Acta Pathol Microbiol Scand A* 1980;88:59-60.

Linell F, Ljungberg O, Andersson I. Breast carcinoma. Aspects of early stages, progression and related problems. *Acta Pathol Microbiol Scand A Suppl* 1980;272:1-233.

MacErlean DP, Nathan BE. Calcification in sclerosing adenosis simulating malignant breast calcification. *Br J Radiol* 1972;45:944-945.

Markey BA, Oberman HA. Non-invasive carcinoma arising in adenosis. *Mod Pathol* 1990;3:63A.

Merino MJ, Llombart-Bosch A, Monteagudo C. Malignant changes associated with sclerosing adenosis. A morphologic and immunohistochemical analysis of seven cases. *Mod Pathol* 1990;3:66A.

McDivitt RW, Boyce W, Gersell D. Tubular carcinoma of the breast. Clinical and pathological observations concerning 135 cases. *Am J Surg Pathol* 1982;6:401-411.

58   Nielsen BD. Adenosis tumor of the breast. A clinicopathological investigation of 27 cases. *Histopathology* 1987;11:1259-1275.

Nielsen M, Christensen L, Andersen JA. Radial scars in women with breast cancer. *Cancer* 1987;59:1019-1025.

Nielsen M, Jensen J, Andersen JA. An autopsy study of radial scar in the female breast. *Histopathology* 1985;9:287-295.

Page DL, Anderson TJ. *Diagnostic Histopathology of the Breast*. Churchill Livingstone, Edinburgh, 1987, p 89.

Rickert RR, Kalisher L, Hutter RVP. Indurative mastopathy. A benign sclerosing lesion of breast with elastosis which may simulate carcinoma. *Cancer* 1981;47:561-571.

Rosen PP. Microglandular adenosis. A benign lesion simulating invasive mammary carcinoma. *Am J Surg Pathol* 1983;7:137-144.

Rosenblum MK, Purrazzella R, Rosen PP. Is microglandular adenosis a precancerous disease? A study of carcinoma arising therein. *Am J Surg Pathol* 1986;10:237-245.

Simpson JF, Page DL, DuPont WD. Apocrine adenosis. An occasional mimicker of breast carcinoma. *Mod Pathol* 1990;3:53A.

Tanaka Y, Oota K. A stereomicroscopic study of the mastopathic human breast. I. Three-dimensional structures of abnormal duct evolution and their histologic entity. *Virchows Arch A* 1970;349:195-214.

Tanaka Y, Oota K. A stereomicroscopic study of the mastopathic human breast. II. Three-dimensional structures of abnormal duct evolution and their histologic entity. *Virchows Arch A* 1970;349:215-228.

Tavassoli FA, Norris HJ. Microglandular adenosis of the breast. A clinicopathologic study of 11 cases with ultrastructural observations. *Am J Surg Pathol* 1983;7:731-737.

Taylor HB, Norris HJ. Epithelial invasion of nerves in benign diseases of the breast. *Cancer* 1967; 20:2245-2249.

Tremblay G, Buell RH, Seemayer TA. Elastosis in benign sclerosing ductal proliferation of the female breast. *Am J Surg Pathol* 1977;1:155-159.

Wellings SR, Alpers CE. Subgross pathologic features and incidence of radial scars in the breast. *Hum Pathol* 1984;15:475-479.

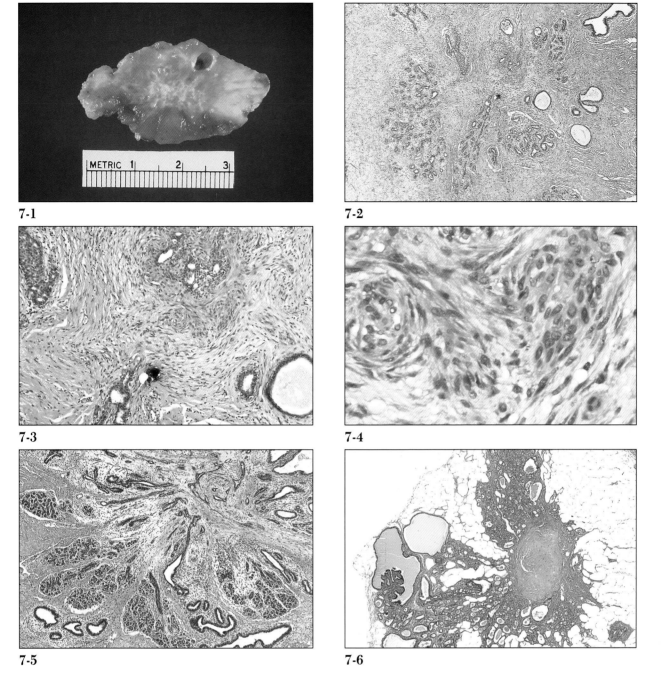

7-1

7-2

7-3

7-4

7-5

7-6

Figure 7-1. The gross appearance of a radial scar is indistinguishable from that of a small infiltrating carcinoma. Note the chalky streaks in the center of the scar.

Figure 7-3. A higher magnification of Figure 7-2 shows hypercellular fibrous tissue with more prominent collagen at the periphery of the cellular zone.

Figure 7-5. This better-developed radial scar has more prominent central collagen (upper right). Ductules entrapped in the scar are distorted.

Figure 7-2. The earliest change in a developing radial scar is, presumably, a proliferation of intralobular and interlobular myofibroblasts.

Figure 7-4. Still higher magnification of Figure 7-3 shows plump fibroblastic nuclei with minimal atypia. Very little collagen is present in this region.

Figure 7-6. This small radial scar has a densely elastotic central zone. Most of the epithelium resembles sclerosing adenosis. The small papilloma at left is a rare finding in association with radial scar.

RADIAL SCAR AND ADENOSIS

60

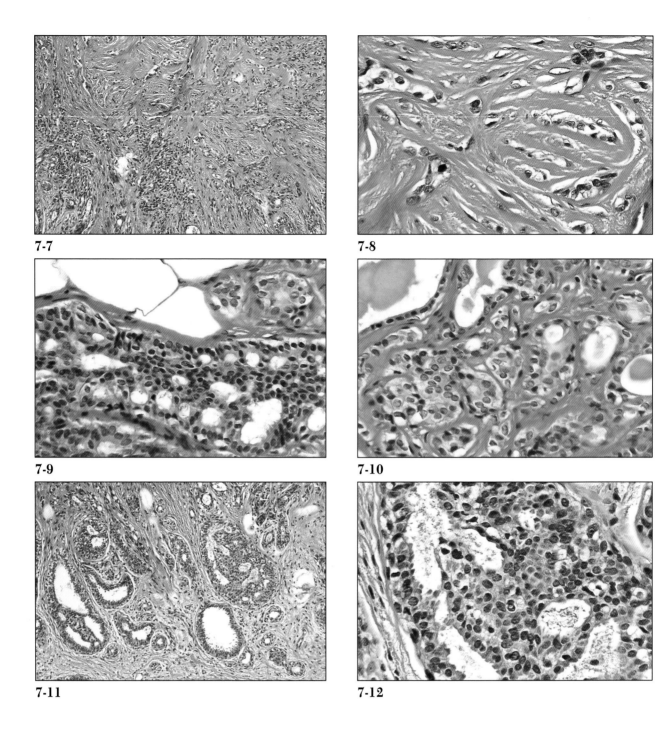

7-7

7-8

7-9

7-10

7-11

7-12

Figure 7-7. The central fibrotic area of this radial scar contains randomly arranged epithelial cells, mimicking infiltrating carcinoma.

Figure 7-9. Proliferating epithelium in radial scar may be hyperplasia of the usual type (pages 92 and 93).

Figure 7-11. Peripheral ductules in radial scar are often the largest in the lesion and may show intraductal hyperplasia.

Figure 7-8. A higher magnification of Figure 7-7 emphasizes the occasionally striking resemblance of radial scar to infiltrating carcinoma.

Figure 7-10. Sclerosing adenosis-like epithelial proliferations are common in radial scar.

Figure 7-12. This example of usual type hyperplasia (pages 92 and 93) in radial scar exhibits the nuclear variability characteristic of this lesion.

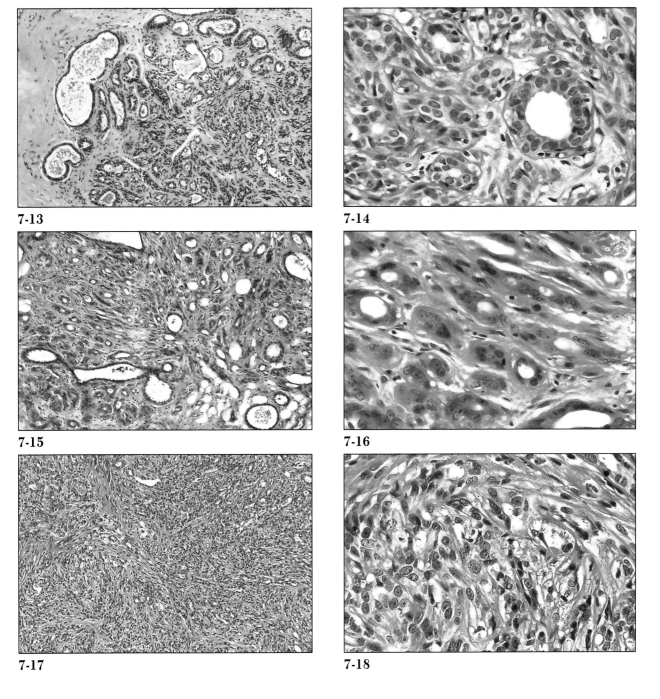

7-13

7-14

7-15

7-16

7-17

7-18

Figure 7-13. The peripherally located ductules of sclerosing adenosis (left and top) tend to have larger diameters than those located centrally (lower right).

Figure 7-15. In some foci, sclerosing adenosis may consist of cords of cells without lumen formation.

Figure 7-17. Sclerosing adenosis may have extremely cellular areas with only rare lumina. Individual lobules are no longer apparent, and this illustration may represent several confluent lobules.

Figure 7-14. Ductules in sclerosing adenosis may form obvious lumina of varying sizes. Other ductules appear as aggregates of cells with small or barely discernible lumina. Only the larger ductules have a clearly recognizable myoepithelial cell layer.

Figure 7-16. Cytologic variation in sclerosing adenosis includes small nuclei and larger, vesicular forms. Nuclei may be ovoid or even spindle-shaped.

Figure 7-18. A higher magnification of Figure 7-17 shows closely packed cells with mild nuclear pleomorphism. Although epithelial and myoepithelial components are probably present, they cannot be distinguished on H&E-stained sections.

62

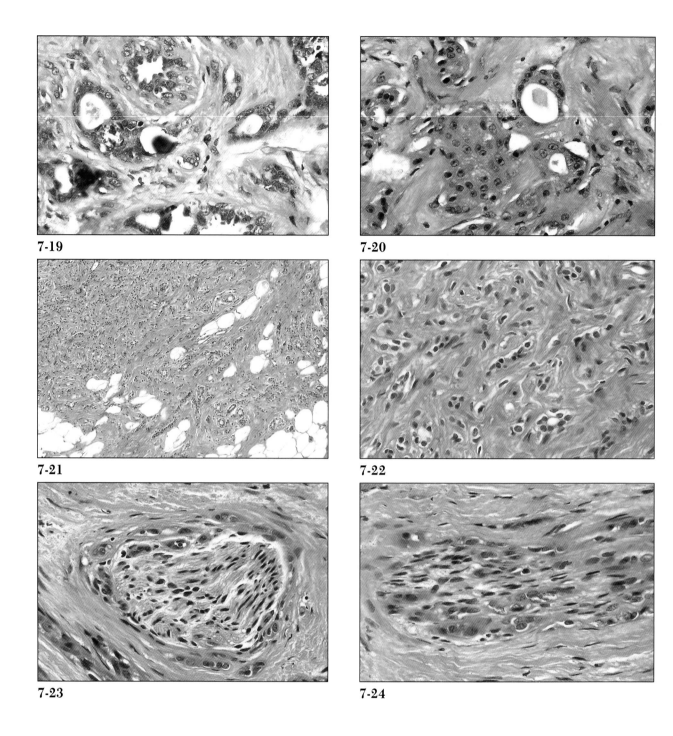

7-19

7-20

7-21

7-22

7-23

7-24

Figure 7-19. This example of sclerosing adenosis exhibits a prominent fibrous stromal component separating the epithelial elements. Intraluminal calcifications are also present and were seen radiographically, leading to a clinical diagnosis of probable carcinoma.

Figure 7-21. This example of sclerosing adenosis from an elderly woman is hypocellular with dense stroma. Only a few lumina are visible. We believe that this represents atrophic change in what was once, presumably, a more cellular proliferation.

Figure 7-23. Sclerosing adenosis may involve the perineural space. In this example, the benign epithelial cells completely encircle the nerve.

Figure 7-20. Apocrine metaplasia may be present in sclerosing adenosis. The enlarged, somewhat pleomorphic nuclei with prominent nucleoli are typical of this metaplastic change wherever it occurs.

Figure 7-22. A higher magnification of Figure 7-21 shows disorganized cords of cells, raising the possibility of infiltrating lobular carcinoma. The many ovoid nuclei seen in this illustration are not a feature of infiltrating lobular carcinoma, however.

Figure 7-24. Probably because of tangential sectioning, the cells of sclerosing adenosis may rarely appear to invade a nerve. In this example, some of the "invading" cells have an apocrine appearance.

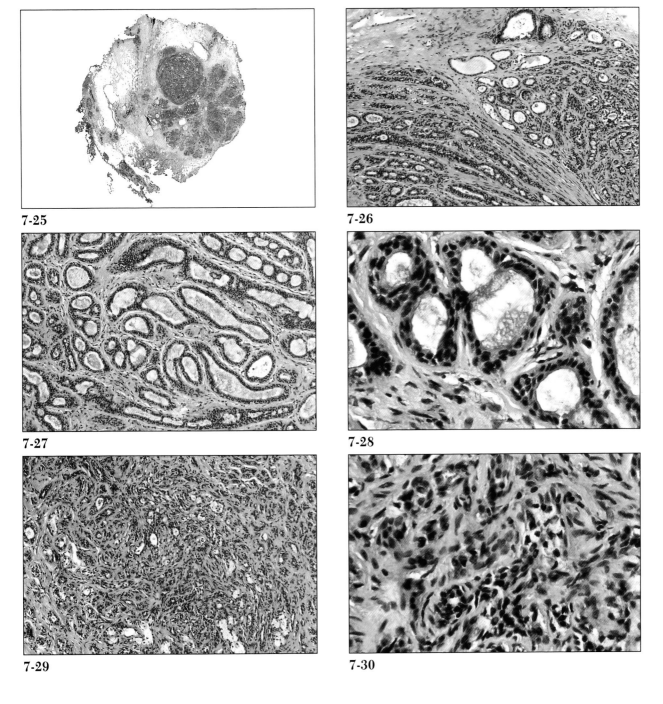

7-25

7-26

7-27

7-28

7-29

7-30

Figure 7-25. This adenosis tumor formed a mammographically detected lesion. The resected mass consists of closely approximated nodules of sclerosing adenosis.

Figure 7-27. Adenosis tumor may have well-formed lumina, including some that are larger than normal ductules.

Figure 7-29. Adenosis tumor may consist of disorganized cells with few lumina. The potential to confuse this mass-forming lesion with carcinoma on frozen sections is obvious.

Figure 7-26. Another example of adenosis tumor forms elongated ductules and cords of cells identical to those seen in sclerosing adenosis. As in the latter lesion, dilated ductules are present peripherally.

Figure 7-28. A higher magnification of Figure 7-27 shows lumina lined by cytologically bland cells. A two-cell layer is visible focally.

Figure 7-30. A higher magnification of Figure 7-29 shows haphazardly arranged but cytologically bland cells, some with spindled nuclei.

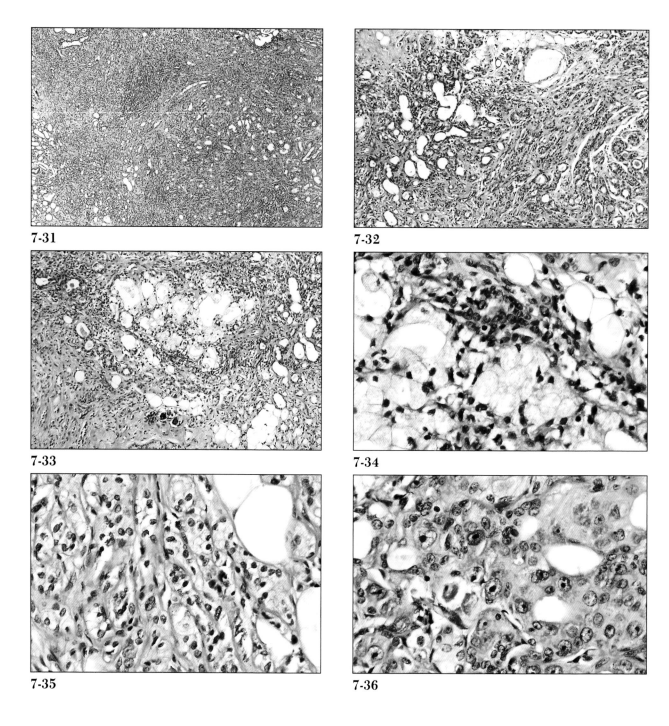

7-31

7-32

7-33

7-34

7-35

7-36

Figure 7-31. This example of adenosis tumor contains both well-formed ductules (right) and more solid areas (upper left).

Figure 7-33. Otherwise typical adenosis tumors may contain foci of clear cell change (page 6).

Figure 7-35. Clear cell change in adenosis tumors may also involve cords of cells lacking lumina. Enlarged, pleomorphic nuclei are evident here, in contrast to the small nuclei seen in Figure 7-34.

Figure 7-32. A higher magnification of Figure 7-31 emphasizes the juxtaposition of well-formed lumina with nests and cords of cells lacking lumina.

Figure 7-34. A higher magnification of Figure 7-33 demonstrates the small, dense nuclei of the clear cells. Entrapped adipose tissue may also be seen in adenosis tumor (upper right).

Figure 7-36. Apocrine metaplasia may involve adenosis tumor, as well as sclerosing adenosis (Figure 7-20). The typical nuclear changes of apocrine cells should not be confused with carcinoma.

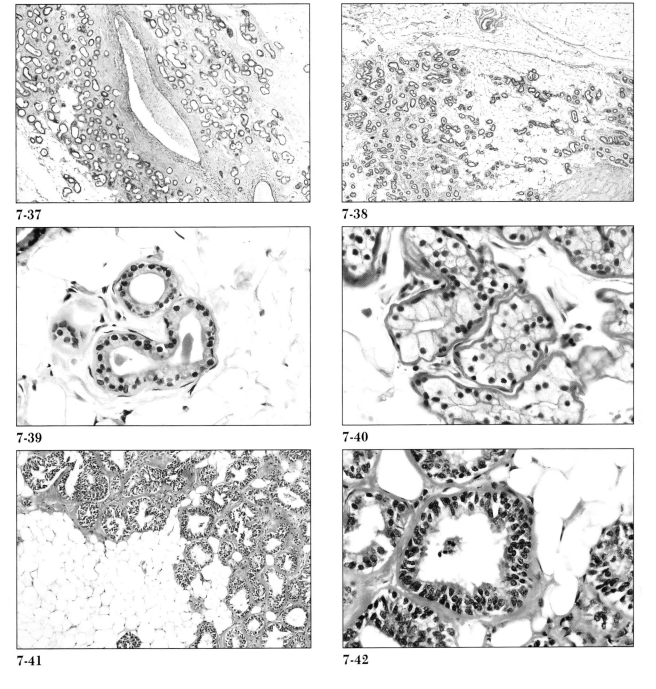

7-37

7-38

7-39

7-40

7-41

7-42

Figure 7-37. Small ductule-like structures are irregularly distributed around a large, sub-segmental duct. Although many of the lumina are circular, others have more variable shapes.

Figure 7-39. The ductule-like structures may be round or slightly elongated. The lining is most often composed of a single layer of uniform cells. Dense luminal secretions, as seen here, are commonly present.

Figure 7-41. Microglandular adenosis may have atypical epithelial cells that are stratified and form irregular intraluminal projections.

Figure 7-38. Ductule-like structures are haphazardly arranged in fat without any evidence of lobule formation.

Figure 7-40. The cells of microglandular adenosis may have voluminous pale to clear cytoplasm that encroaches on the lumen. The nuclei, however, are small and uniform.

Figure 7-42. A higher magnification of Figure 7-41 demonstrates atypical epithelial cells with increased nuclear-to-cytoplasmic ratios and moderate nuclear pleomorphism.

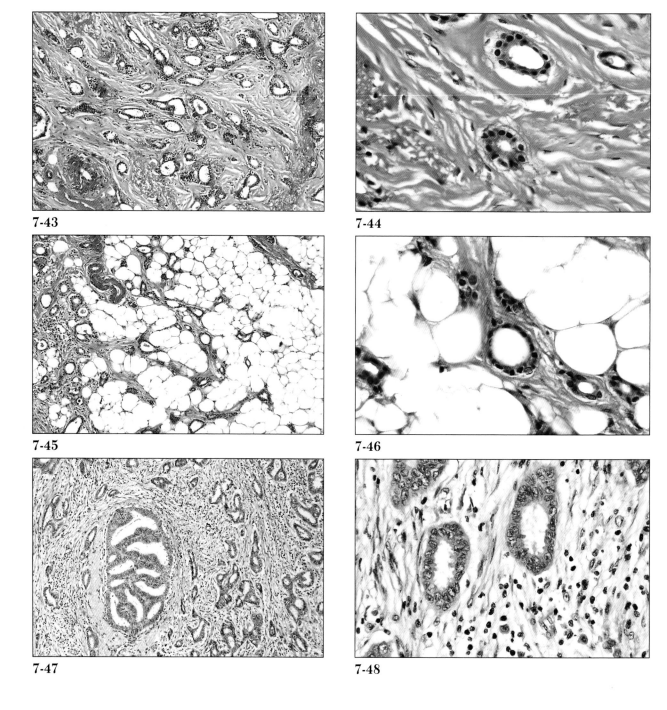

7-43

7-44

7-45

7-46

7-47

7-48

Figure 7-43. Tubular carcinoma has ductule-like structures similar in size to those of microglandular adenosis. Many of the spaces, however, are ovoid or sharply angulated. Microglandular adenosis, in contrast, has ductule-like structures with smoother contours.

Figure 7-45. The periphery of the tubular carcinoma seen in Figures 7-43 and 7-44 has not stimulated a well-defined desmoplastic response.

Figure 7-47. Ductal carcinoma in situ (left center) is associated with an infiltrating component that forms ductule-like structures. However, the latter structures demonstrate epithelial bridging (right), unlike microglandular adenosis.

Figure 7-44. The ductule-like structures of tubular carcinoma are frequently composed of cells with apocrine "snouts." Note the marked desmoplasia, in contrast with microglandular adenosis.

Figure 7-46. A higher magnification of Figure 7-45 shows cells with eosinophilic cytoplasm typical of tubular carcinoma.

Figure 7-48. Higher magnification of Figure 7-47 shows conspicuous nuclear abnormalities in the epithelial cells, including a high nuclear-to-cytoplasmic ratio. These abnormalities separate this lesion from both tubular carcinoma and microglandular adenosis.

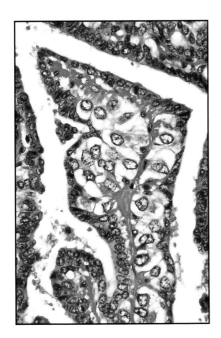

8

PAPILLOMAS, DUCTAL ADENOMAS, AND ADENOMYOEPITHELIOMAS

The three benign entities discussed together in this section share several microscopic features and often have overlapping appearances. Intraductal papillomas may be found in both small and large ducts. Some benign intraductal proliferations, with or without a papillary architecture, include a prominent myoepithelial component, and lesions of the latter type have been referred to *adenomyoepitheliomas*.

MULTIPLE PAPILLOMAS OF SMALL DUCTS

Papillomas differ from hyperplasia by having fibrovascular cores. They involve subsegmental small ducts deep in the substance of the breast. The smallest papillomas can be seen to arise from dilated ductules in unfolding lobules (Figures 8-1, 8-2). In contrast to the solitary papillomas of the large ducts, discussed in the next section, papillomas of small ducts are usually multiple (Figures 8-3, 8-4). Azzopardi estimated that papillomas of small ducts are only one tenth as common as the solitary papillomas of large ducts. The term *papillomatosis* has frequently been used for multiple papillomas of small ducts. As noted above, this term has also been used to denote

multiple ducts involved by ordinary hyperplasia. Because of this confusion, we prefer to avoid the term completely and substitute the designation of *multiple papillomas*. If the term papillomatosis is used, its meaning should be clearly specified.

Whether patients with multiple papillomas are at increased risk for subsequent invasive carcinoma is difficult to ascertain. The frequent association of hyperplasia of the usual type, with small duct papillomas, makes it difficult to judge whether multiple papillomas are an independent variable. Carter found that two of six patients with multiple papillomas subsequently developed carcinoma, whereas two of 14 patients who had multiple papillomas plus hyperplasia of the usual type developed carcinoma. Haagensen reported that six of 52 patients with multiple papillomas developed carcinoma. In the latter series, the patients had been followed up for an average of 19 years and the average interval between excision of the papillomas and the development of carcinoma was 17 years. There is no calculated statistical risk for a comparable population of patients. It is also unclear whether other forms of hyperplasia were present. Currently, it seems reasonable to view papillomas of the small ducts as a manifestation of epithelial hyperplasia of the usual type. This places the patient at a slightly in-

68 creased risk (1.5 to two times) for carcinoma as compared with the population at large (Hutter).

In the smallest papillomas, the stroma may be only a single capillary with a negligible cuff of collagen. It is often cut in cross section and is barely discernible. The epithelial cells display a spectrum of appearances similar to the variation seen in large papillomas. There may be a single layer of epithelial cells with a variable number of myoepithelial cells or more complex tubular arrangements of the epithelium. Papillomas in small ducts are accompanied frequently by fibrocystic changes, and it is those fibrocystic changes that produce a clinically palpable mass. Small papillomas may contribute to a palpable abnormality, but they are not palpable by themselves.

The meticulous three-dimensional reconstruction study by Ohuchi et al demonstrated that multiple small duct papillomas always originate in the terminal duct–lobular unit. This is also the site of hyperplasia, and the simultaneous occurrence of hyperplasia and papillomatosis in a microscopic section is thus not surprising. Ohuchi et al also demonstrated that a duct system containing multiple small papillomas could have multiple foci of ductal carcinoma in situ. A similar observation has been made by Papotti et al. When these foci of atypical cells form solid aggregates and consist of a monomorphic population of round cells with sharp borders, they resemble the cells of lobular carcinoma in situ (Figures 8-5, 8-6). We also view such foci as a manifestation of ductal carcinoma in situ. Given the origin of small duct papillomas from the terminal duct–lobular unit as described above, it is not surprising that a mixture of papilloma and ductal carcinoma could occur in the same duct.

The presence, focally, of an abnormal monomorphic population of cells in an otherwise typical papilloma produces a difficult diagnostic problem. One can interpret this as a papilloma with focal ductal carcinoma in situ or diagnose the lesion as atypical papilloma in which the basis for the atypia is a cytologically distinct population of abnormal cells that only partially involves a duct. The risk for subsequent invasive carcinoma is not known for this combination. Presumably, it lies between that of a papilloma and fully diagnostic ductal carcinoma in situ. At the very least, the presence of such foci should stimulate a search for ducts that are completely involved with such cells and thus fully diag-nostic of carcinoma in situ. All of the tissue should be submitted for examination when a biopsy specimen contains an atypical papilloma. Whatever term is used, the surgeon should understand the "gray zone" encompassed by such a lesion. The range of risk for subsequent invasive cancer, even if not precise, can still be conveyed.

SOLITARY LARGE DUCT PAPILLOMA

Solitary papillomas of the large ducts are manifested by nipple discharge in about 75% of cases. The remainder are typically found by palpation. Papillomas can occur in any decade of life, but 60% of patients are 35 to 55 years old, and most of the remainder are beyond 55 years of age (Haagensen).

Grossly, papillomas of the large ducts range from 1 or 2 mm to up to 3 cm in diameter. The smaller lesions may be barely discernible on gross examination, and occasionally are found only by blocking and sectioning the entire specimen. Grossly visible papillomas are tan or red with a convoluted external surface (Figure 8-7). Papillomas are usually soft and friable, but may be firm because of a large component of fibrous tissue.

The low-power pattern is extremely variable, depending on the relative quantity and arrangement of the fibrovascular connective tissue (Figure 8-8). The epithelium may vary from a single cell lining to hyperplasia. In a given area, epithelium or stroma can dominate. The epithelial component of papillomas is histologically and cytologically diverse. It may be identical to that of normal ducts, with evenly spaced, cuboidal or low columnar eosinophilic epithelial cells overlying a well-defined layer of myoepithelial cells. Often the epithelium is columnar, with elongated nuclei and a pseudostratified appearance (Figure 8-9). Sometimes the cells are small with dense nuclei (Figure 8-10). A mild to modest degree of nuclear pleomorphism is common (Figure 8-11). In other foci, nuclei may be vesicular (Figure 8-12). Apocrine metaplasia is occasionally seen (Figure 8-13). When the cytoplasm is scant, the nuclei may appear to be immediately juxtaposed (Figure 8-14) or overlap (Figure 8-15). There may be focal areas of epithelial "tufting" (Figure 8-16). The myoepithelial layer is often invisible, at least by light microscopy, and this should never be used as a criterion for discarding the diagnosis of papilloma. On the other hand, myoepithelial cells may appear prominent when they are numerous or cut tangentially (Figure 8-12).

The fibrovascular stalks of papillomas vary in their amount of fibrous tissue and capillary size. It is common for larger papillomas to have dense deposits of sparsely cellular or acellular collagen. This probably occurs secondary to epithelial necrosis with replacement of epithelium and capillaries by collagen. Much of a papilloma may be hyalinized, especially one that occurs in a large duct. This leads to an irregular arrangement of the residual epithelium that may cause concern because the overall pattern of the papilloma is lost. The cells are cytologically bland, however, thereby differing from carcinoma.

The wall of the involved duct may be thickened and fibrotic or it may be only a thin rim. The more fibrotic walls often contain entrapped epithelium (Figure 8-17). This probably represents hyalinization and fibrosis of the peripheral portion of a papilloma. The cells within the fibrotic wall are cytologically identical to those of the papilloma, thus allowing the distinction from an invasive carcinoma (Figure 8-18).

Murad et al noted infarcted areas in 17% of papillomas. Sometimes, the infarction is extensive, but the structure of the preexistent papilloma is usually discernible (Figure 8-19). Degenerating epithelial and stromal cells are irregularly arranged (Figure 8-20). There may be, however, a fibrous tissue response that distorts the papilloma and results in entrapped epithelium (Figures 8-21, 8-22). The resultant appearance is similar to that of sclerosing adenosis (Murad et al). The entrapped epithelium usually lacks the pattern of the associated papilloma, but it has no cytologic atypia. In effect, one can apply the same approach to entrapped epithelium in infarcted papillomas as is used for epithelium in the duct wall of papillomas described above. Infarcted papillomas also may have squamous metaplasia that is intermixed with a fibrous tissue response, yielding a haphazard arrangement that mimics squamous cell carcinoma (Figures 8-23, 8-24). The diagnosis of squamous carcinoma can be avoided by recognizing that the squamous cells are within a duct and that there are remnants of intact or necrotic papilloma.

Papillomas may be partially involved by carcinoma that is cytologically and architecturally identical to various types of ductal carcinoma in situ. The distinction of papilloma from papillary carcinoma rests on the cytologic features of the epithelium. By definition, papillomas and papillary carcinoma share a low-power morphology determined by the presence of fibrovascular stalks supporting the epithelium. As discussed in the section on ductal carcinoma in situ, the various subtypes of this neoplasm can occur on fibrovascular stalks. Thus, there may be large, pleomorphic cells with necrosis, typical of comedocarcinoma, or there may be micropapillary and cribriform proliferations identical to those variants of ductal carcinoma in situ that lack fibrovascular cores.

Papillomas may be only focally involved by carcinoma, with large areas having a typical, benign appearance (Figures 8-25 to 8-36). The carcinoma is usually a cytologically distinct population that may consist of large apocrine-like cells (Figures 8-27 to 8-30) or monomorphic cells with lightly staining nuclei. Mitotic figures are often prominent in such areas and may be atypical (Figure 8-30). In other lesions, the malignant cells have scant cytoplasm (Figures 8-34 to 8-36). Perhaps the most easily overlooked form of papillary carcinoma associated with a papilloma is the type characterized by elongated epithelial cells arranged perpendicular to the connective tissue stalk. These cells often have small amounts of cytoplasm, and elongated, stratified, but uniformly hyperchromatic nuclei. Papillary carcinoma is described in greater detail in the section on page 114.

DUCTAL ADENOMA

Ductal adenoma, as currently defined, is a morphologically heterogeneous group of predominately solid (noncystic) lesions characterized by epithelial and stromal proliferation, usually surrounded by a rim of fibrous tissue. We agree with Page and Anderson, who have referred to ductal adenomas as "muddling lesions of which the nature and confines of definition are not clear." The term is useful, however, to acknowledge a proliferation that does not fall into other well-recognized categories. Many microscopic features of so-called adenomyoepithelioma of the breast overlap with those of ductal adenoma. Thus, the classification of predominantly solid intraductal epithelial and stromal proliferations may be arbitrary. At the moment it does not appear to be necessary to sharply separate ductal adenomas and myoepitheliomas, but we should be careful to recognize that both are benign. Nevertheless, because the literature implies that these are separate entities, we will discuss ductal adenomas and adenomyoepitheliomas as if they were truly distinct lesions.

Azzopardi and Salm first applied the term ductal adenoma to an epithelial and stromal proliferation that fills small and medium-sized ducts. None of the 24 cases reported by Azzopardi and Salm arose in large subareolar ducts. However, lesions diagnosed as ductal adenoma by Lammie and Millis were frequently found in major ducts and formed a palpable mass near the nipple. More than half of the adenomas reported by Azzopardi and Salm were multiple, as opposed to only one of 14 cases in the series by Lammie and Millis. It is likely, as will be described below, that differences in the classification of ductal adenomas vis-á-vis ductal papillomas account for these variations.

Women with ductal adenomas have ranged from 20 to 77 years of age, but more than 80% have been over 40 years old, and 50% of the patients described by Lammie and Millis were over 60 years old. Palpable lesions have always been reported to be unilateral and have been present for durations ranging from several weeks to several years. Nipple discharge is seen occasionally in patients with a palpable lesion near the nipple. Nonpalpable adenomas may be detected mammographically, especially when calcified. Ductal adenomas may be associated with fibrocystic changes elsewhere in the breast, including sclerosing adenosis, epithelial hyperplasia, and cysts. Azzopardi and Salm, as well as Lammie and Millis, have noted an association with duct ectasia.

In the series by Azzopardi and Salm, two biopsy specimens contained coexistent, noninvasive carcinoma that was topographically unrelated to the adenoma. The patients were 56 and 60 years old; one had lobular carcinoma in situ and the other had ductal carcinoma in situ. In the families of patients with ductal adenoma there has been no increase in the frequency of breast cancer and follow-up has been uneventful.

Ductal adenomas vary from 0.2 to 3 cm in size. Grossly, they are sharply defined, gray or white nodules that may have a gritty consistency on their cut surfaces, depending on the amount of fibrous tissue and calcium. Ductal adenomas may be indistinguishable from infiltrating carcinoma if the central area is densely fibrotic (see below).

The microscopic appearance of ductal adenoma is extraordinarily variable. The center of the adenoma may be densely fibrotic, scarlike, and devoid of epithelium (Figure 8-37). Irregular deposits of calcium are sometimes seen in the central portion of the lesion and, less often, at the periphery. Conversely, the glandular elements may be concentrated in the center of the mass, with the fibrous areas closer to the periphery. Many ductal adenomas contain focal lymphocytic infiltrates and, rarely, germinal centers.

The periphery of ductal adenoma is almost always surrounded by a distinct fibrous rim (Figure 8-38), but rarely the epithelium directly abuts adipose tissue. Occasionally, irregular nests of epithelium become enmeshed within the fibrous tissue rim of ductal adenoma. Such areas suggest the presence of a carcinoma with capsular invasion (Figure 8-39). The cytologic features of the cells and the architectural resemblance of these entrapped nests to the intraductal component should deter the diagnosis of malignancy (Figure 8-40).

The epithelium of ductal adenoma is a mixture of myoepithelial and epithelial cells. The latter component frequently has apocrine features, with characteristic large nuclei and prominent nucleoli (Figure 8-41). Mitotic figures are usually rare, but Azzopardi and Salm found as many as eight per 20 high-power fields in one case. The epithelial elements may form well-defined, small ductules (Figure 8-42). In other foci, the ductules may be contiguous, distorted, and have less obvious lumina, resembling sclerosing adenosis (Figure 8-43). There may be a mixture of patterns with sclerosing adenosis-like areas, papilloma-like areas, and densely sclerotic foci (Figures 8-44 to 8-46). These may occur in different regions of the same lesion, suggesting that multiple, closely associated ducts have been altered and become confluent. Only rarely are ductal adenomas clearly multifocal, with large areas of uninvolved breast tissue between them.

Intraductal papillomas contain solid areas that are microscopically identical to ductal adenomas. It seems likely that, in many instances, the solid proliferations of ductal adenoma are intraductal papillomas that have lost their papillary architecture as the stroma and epithelium proliferate to fill the duct (Figures 8-47, 8-48).

ADENOMYOEPITHELIOMA

Adenomyoepitheliomas are a morphologically heterogenous group of tumors with a conspicuous component of myoepithelial cells intermixed with epithelium-lined lumina (Figures 8-49, 8-50). The special appellation of adenomyoepithelioma has been reserved for lesions that not only have a large number of periductal myoepithelial cells, but also possess a prominent stromal component of spindle-shaped cells. The latter are also believed to have myoepithelial features.

Adenomyoepitheliomas occur in women from 27 to 80 years old and may present as a palpable mass or be identified mammographically. Others are microscopic findings involving multiple ducts (Toth). Clinically detectable adenomyoepitheliomas are well-circumscribed, firm masses measuring up to 2.5 cm in diameter. The cut surface may be tan, gray, or white. The varied coloration undoubtedly reflects the microscopic heterogeneity of the group.

The spectrum of microscopic findings is broad, both architecturally and cytologically. The tumor may be multinodular with areas of confluence, or it may be a single nodule. Adenomyoepitheliomas can have the low-power pattern of a papilloma (Figure 8-51). The nodular and papillary patterns are frequently intermixed, and may be associated with central fibrotic zones. The focal papillary pattern and central fibrotic fibrosis are features shared with ductal adenomas.

Many myoepithelial cells in adenomyoepithelioma are round or polyhedral and have almost clear cytoplasm (Figure 8-52). Their cytoplasm allows for ready distinction on H&E-stained sections from more darkly staining epithelial cells. The relatively clear myoepithelial cells are part of a continuous spectrum of myoepithelial-type cells that also includes elongated cells lacking distinct cell borders (Figure 8-53). Round, spindled, or intermediately shaped myoepithelial cells often form broad sheets in these neoplasms. Mitotic figures are occasionally seen in the myoepithelial cell component.

As the name implies, there is also an epithelial component in adenomyoepithelioma that is intimately intermixed with the myoepithelial population. The epithelium may consist of well-formed ductules surrounded by sheets of myoepithelial cells. In some foci, the ductules are distinct and identical to those seen in ductal adenoma (Figure 8-54). In complex papillomatous areas, however, the epithelial cells assume correspondingly more irregular configurations.

Several reported cases of adenomyoepithelioma have had either a minor or major infiltrating component resembling microglandular adenosis. These areas consist of small, round, gland-like spaces lined with a double layer of epithelium. The innermost epithelial layer has been viewed as having apocrine features by some authors (Eusebi et al). The myoepithelial layer may consist of normal-appearing myoepithelial cells or large cells resembling those described in the section on clear cell change. The term adenomyoepithelial adenosis has been used for this infiltrating lesion (Kiaer et al). Local recurrence has been associated with this infiltrating pattern (Kiaer et al, Young and Clement).

Pure myoepithelial proliferations have been reported that were not circumscribed or confined to ducts (Erlandson and Rosen, Bigotti and DiGiorgio). Whether these infiltrating myoepitheliomas are related to well-circumscribed adenomyoepitheliomas is uncertain. Ducts may be found within the infiltrating component, but are probably entrapped by the myoepithelial proliferation and are not an intrinsic part of the lesion, as is the case in adenomyoepithelioma. One case of infiltrating myoepithelioma had a lymph node metastasis (Thorner et al).

REFERENCES

Azzopardi JG. *Problems in Breast Pathology.* Philadelphia, WB Saunders Co, 1979, pp 151, 164-165.

Azzopardi JG, Salm R. Ductal adenoma of the breast. A lesion which can mimic carcinoma. *J Pathol* 1984;144:15-23.

Bigotti G, DiGiorgio CG. Myoepithelioma of the breast. Histologic, immunologic and electronmicroscopic appearance. *J Surg Oncol* 1986;32:58-64.

Carter D. Intraductal papillary tumors of the breast. A study of 78 cases. *Cancer* 1977;39: 1689-1692.

Erlandson RA, Rosen PP. Infiltrating myoepithelioma of the breast. *Am J Surg Pathol* 1982;6:785-793.

Eusebi V, Casadei GP, Bussolati G, Azzopardi JG. Adenomyoepithelioma of the breast with a distinctive type of apocrine adenosis. *Histopathology* 1987;11:305-315.

Flint A, Oberman HA. Infarction and squamous metaplasia of intraductal papilloma. A benign breast lesion that may simulate carcinoma. *Hum Pathol* 1984;15:764-767.

Gusterson BA, Sloane JP, Middwood C, et al. Ductal adenoma of the breast. A lesion exhibiting a myoepithelial/epithelial phenotype. *Histopathology* 1987;11:103-110.

72 Haagensen CD. *Diseases of the Breast*, ed 3. Philadelphia, WB Saunders Co, 1986, pp 139, 176-191.

Hutter RVP. Consensus statement. Is 'fibrocystic disease' of the breast precancerous? *Arch Pathol Lab Med* 1986;110:171-173.

Jabi M, Dardick I, Cardigos N. Adenomyoepithelioma of the breast. *Arch Pathol Lab Med* 1988;112:73-76.

Kiaer H, Nielsen B, Paulsen S, et al. Adenomyoepithelial adenosis and low-grade malignant adenomyoepithelioma of the breast. *Virchows Arch A* 1984;405:55-67.

Lammie GA, Millis RR. Ductal adenoma of the breast. A review of fifteen cases. *Hum Pathol* 1989;20:903-908.

Murad TM, Contesso G, Mouriesse H. Papillary tumors of large lactiferous ducts. *Cancer* 1981;48:122-133.

Murad TM, Swaid S, Pritchett P. Malignant and benign papillary lesions of the breast. *Hum Pathol* 1977;8:379-390.

Ohuchi N, Abe R, Kasai M. Possible cancerous change of intraductal papillomas of the breast. A 3-D reconstruction study of 25 cases. *Cancer* 1984;54:605-611.

Page DL, Anderson TJ. *Diagnostic Histopathology of the Breast.* Churchill Livingstone, Edinburgh, 1987, p 113.

Papotti M, Gugliotta P, Ghiringhello B, Bussolati G. Association of breast carcinoma and multiple intraductal papillomas. An histological and immunohistochemical investigation. *Histopathology* 1984;8:963-975.

Raju UB, Lee MW, Zarbo RJ, Crissman JD. Papillary neoplasia of the breast. Immunohistochemically defined myoepithelial cells in the diagnosis of benign and malignant papillary breast neoplasms. *Mod Pathol* 1989;2:569-576.

Rosen PP. Papillary duct hyperplasia of the breast in children and young adults. *Cancer* 1985;56:1611-1617.

Rosen PP. Adenomyoepithelioma of the breast. *Hum Pathol* 1987;18:1232-1237.

Thorner PS, Kahn HJ, Baumal R, et al. Malignant myoepithelioma of the breast. An immunohistochemical study by light and electron microscopy. *Cancer* 1986;57:745-750.

Toth J. Benign human mammary myoepithelioma. *Virchows Arch A* 1977;374:263-269.

Weidner N, Levine JD. Spindle-cell adenomyoepithelioma of the breast. A microscopic, ultrastructural, and immunocytochemical study. *Cancer* 1988;62:1561-1567.

Young RH, Clement PB. Adenomyoepithelioma of the breast. A report of three cases and review of the literature. *Am J Clin Pathol* 1988;89:308-314.

Zarbo RJ, Oberman HA. Cellular adenomyoepithelioma of the breast. *Am J Surg Pathol* 1983;7:863-870.

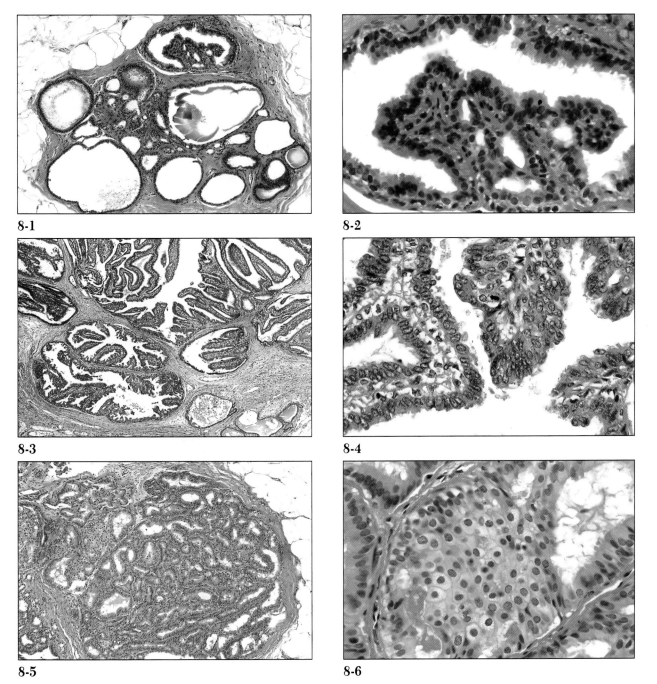

8-1

8-2

8-3

8-4

8-5

8-6

Figure 8-1. An unfolding lobule contains a small intraductal papilloma.

Figure 8-3. When multiple ducts are involved with papillomas, the term *papillomatosis* is often used.

Figure 8-5. This example of atypical papilloma consists of a complex ductal papilloma containing several foci at the left of cytologically atypical cells.

Figure 8-2. A higher magnification of Figure 8-1 discloses a delicate fibrovascular core. This feature distinguishes papillomas from epithelial hyperplasia of the usual type.

Figure 8-4. Some papillomas have conspicuous myoepithelial cells that may, as in this example, have clear cytoplasm. Typical-appearing mitotic figures are occasionally present.

Figure 8-6. A higher magnification of Figure 8-5 shows a monomorphic population of cells with well-defined cytoplasmic borders and powdery eosinophilic cytoplasm. This cell population is in marked contrast to the apocrine epithelium constituting the remainder of the papilloma.

74

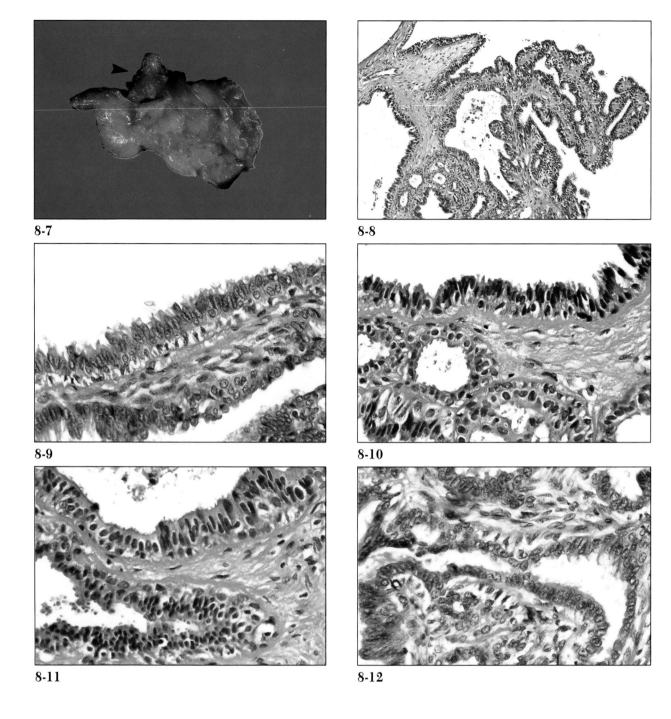

8-7

8-8

8-9

8-10

8-11

8-12

Figure 8-7. An opened large duct contains a papilloma approximately 9 mm in diameter at the top of the specimen (arrow).

Figure 8-9. This fibrovascular stalk has a myoepithelial cell layer that is conspicuous at the top of the stalk and absent at the bottom. The nuclei of the epithelial cell layer are elongated and overlapping and appear pseudostratified.

Figure 8-11. The epithelial cells in this papilloma exhibit moderate nuclear pleomorphism. Most nuclei are ovoid and vary considerably in size; others are spindled. Tangential sectioning may give the epithelium a disorganized appearance (bottom).

Figure 8-8. This large duct papilloma has well-defined, branching fibrovascular stalks. The irregular configuration of the papilloma leads to planes of section that appear to contain entrapped epithelium.

Figure 8-10. Some papillomas contain dense epithelial cell nuclei with scant cytoplasm (top).

Figure 8-12. The epithelial cells of this papilloma have overlapping, vesicular nuclei and scant cytoplasm.

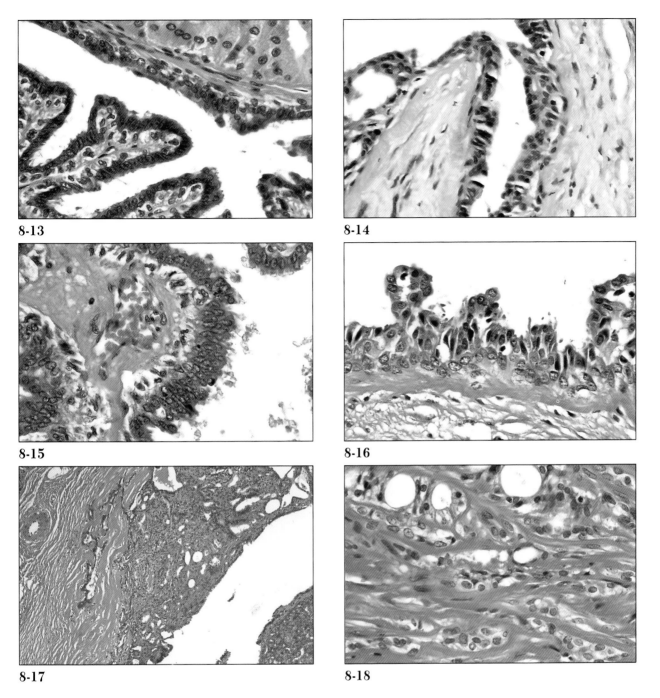

8-13

8-14

8-15

8-16

8-17

8-18

Figure 8-13. Papillomas can have considerable cytologic variation. Apocrine metaplasia is seen (top). Elsewhere, nuclei are either vesicular or dense, with spindle, ovoid, or round shapes.

Figure 8-15. Epithelial cells with high nuclear-to-cytoplasmic ratios have overlapping, stratified nuclei similar to papillary carcinoma. In this particular lesion, the presense of myoepithelial cells can be used as a criterion of benignancy.

Figure 8-17. The fibrous wall at the edge of this papilloma contains entrapped epithelium, raising the possibility of invasion.

Figure 8-14. This papilloma has apparently stratified nuclei exhibiting marked variation in shape. Some nuclei are quite dense and others are more lightly staining.

Figure 8-16. The papilloma has tufting of epithelium. Irregularly shaped, hyperchromatic nuclei are probably in degenerating cells. All of the nuclei, however, are within the spectrum of an ordinary papilloma.

Figure 8-18. A higher magnification from the same case as Figure 8-17 shows entrapped cells with cytologic features identical to those of the associated papilloma.

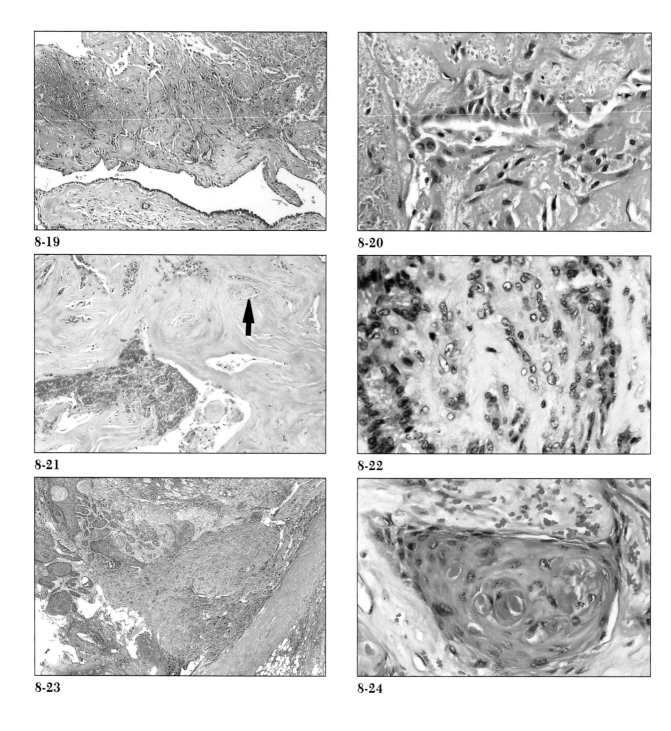

8-19

8-20

8-21

8-22

8-23

8-24

Figure 8-19. This infarcted papilloma retains its fibrovascular stalks, although these have become sclerotic and focally their epithelium is denuded.

Figure 8-21. Infarction of papillomas with patchy epithelial necrosis (arrow) and stromal fibrosis eventually leads to irregular nests of epithelium entrapped in a sclerotic stroma (upper left).

Figure 8-23. This infarcted papilloma has broad areas of fibrosis (right). Large areas of squamous metaplasia are also present.

Figure 8-20. Scattered, degenerating epithelial and stromal cells in an infarcted papilloma may create a haphazard, disorganized image.

Figure 8-22. A higher magnification of entrapped epithelium from another infarcted papilloma shows that the cells lack organization. Nonetheless, the uniform blandness of the nuclei distinguishes these benign cells from carcinoma.

Figure 8-24. The squamous metaplasia contains cells that form keratin pearls and have active-appearing nuclei.

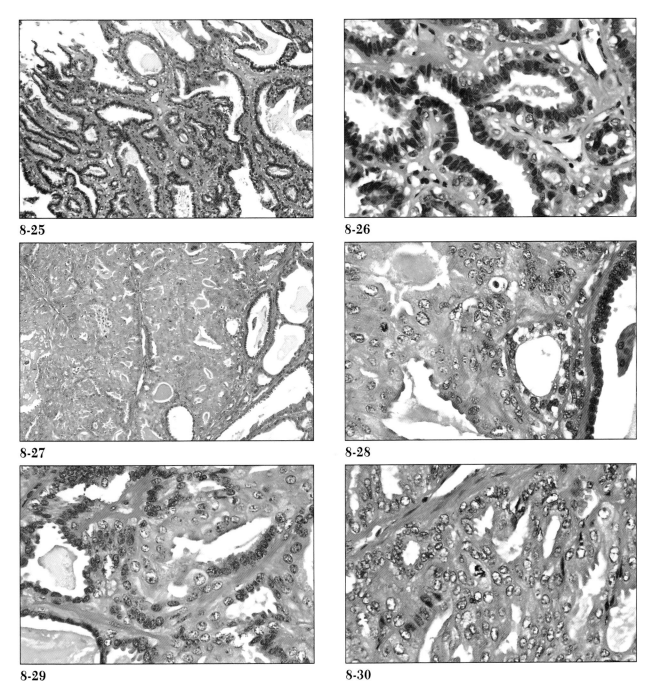

8-25

8-26

8-27

8-28

8-29

8-30

Figure 8-25. Figures 8-25 to 8-30 illustrate a carcinoma arising in a presumably preexistent papilloma. At low magnification this portion of the lesion has the characteristic architectural features of a typical papilloma. However, a few foci of atypical epithelial cells are seen, especially at the top of the lesion.

Figure 8-27. Elsewhere, the papilloma illustrated in Figures 8-25 and 8-26 has broad sheets of atypical cells lacking a papillomatous architecture. The associated papillomatous component is seen at the right.

Figure 8-29. Cytologically benign epithelium of the papilloma is contiguous with the atypical cells at multiple foci.

Figure 8-26. A higher magnification of Figure 8-25 illustrates the myoepithelial and epithelial cells of a typical papilloma.

Figure 8-28. A higher magnification of Figure 8-27 shows the juxtaposition of typical epithelium (right) and markedly atypical cells with enlarged vesicular nuclei (left).

Figure 8-30. The carcinomatous component contains cells with atypical-appearing mitotic figures.

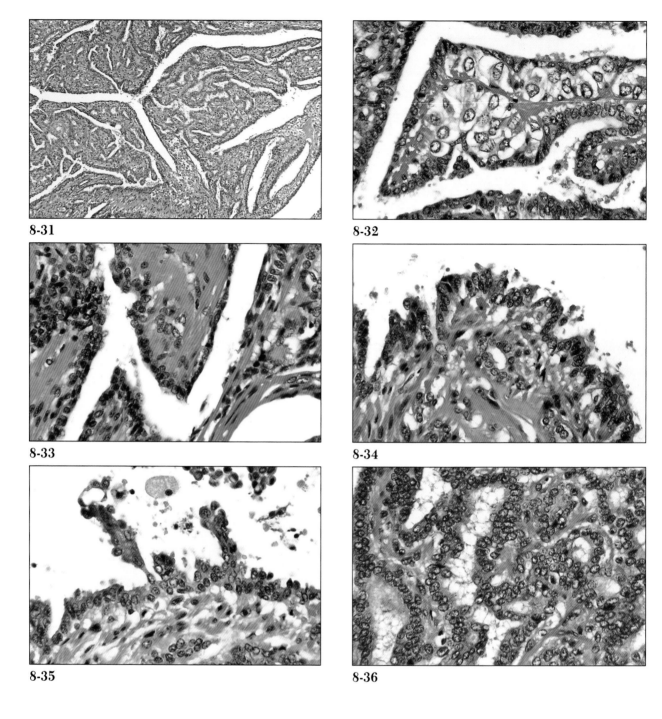

8-31

8-32

8-33

8-34

8-35

8-36

Figure 8-31. Figures 8-31 to 8-36 illustrate another papilloma with focal carcinoma. The typical architecture of a papilloma is present in this field.

Figure 8-33. In some areas the myoepithelial layer is lost, but the epithelial cells are small and benign-appearing.

Figure 8-35. In this focus of severe cytologic atypia, papillae are present. Nuclear and cytoplasmic debris is seen in the lumen. We interpret this as carcinoma.

Figure 8-32. A higher magnification of Figure 8-31 includes epithelium within the spectrum of papilloma, plus prominent myoepithelial cells.

Figure 8-34. In other foci, the epithelium of this papilloma assumes a severely atypical cytologic appearance.

Figure 8-36. These pleomorphic cells have irregularly clumped chromatin and a high nuclear-to-cytoplasmic ratio. This focus of carcinoma maintains a papillary architecture.

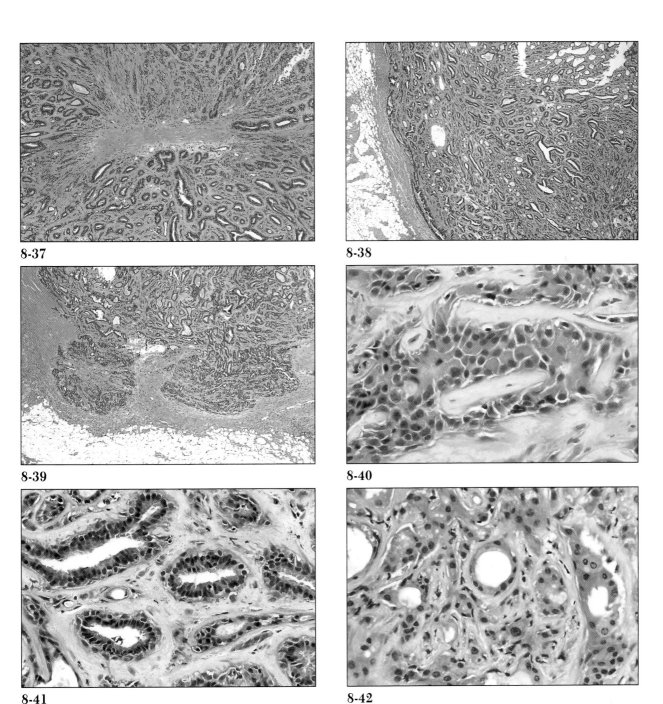

8-37

8-38

8-39

8-40

8-41

8-42

Figure 8-37. The central portion of a ductal adenoma may be sclerotic. The adjacent epithelial components are radially oriented with respect to the central scar.

Figure 8-39. The fibrous rim of ductal adenoma may contain nests and cords of epithelium, mimicking invasion.

Figure 8-41. A well-defined, double layer of cells lines some duct-like structures of ductal adenoma.

Figure 8-38. Ductal adenomas usually have a sharply circumscribed margin with a rim of condensed fibrous tissue. The epithelial component has irregularly shaped ducts of varying size.

Figure 8-40. A higher magnification of Figure 8-39 demonstrates that the "invasive" cells are cytologically bland and identical to the cells of the central portion of the tumor.

Figure 8-42. Apocrine epithelium is frequently present in ductal adenoma. The metaplastic cells may form duct-like structures or be apparently dissociated in the surrounding stroma.

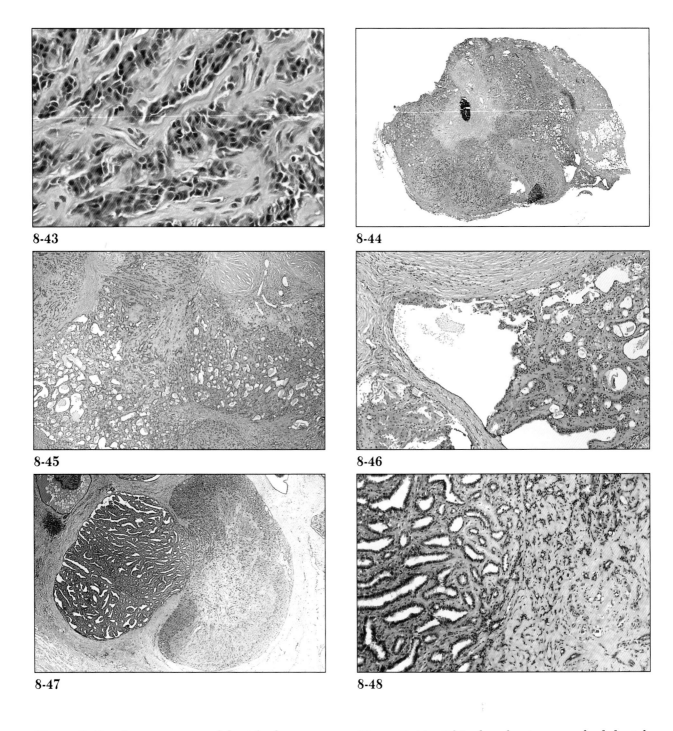

8-43

8-44

8-45

8-46

8-47

8-48

Figure 8-43. In many areas of ductal adenoma, lumina are absent and the cells form irregular cords. This microscopic pattern is similar to some areas of sclerosing adenosis.

Figure 8-45. A higher magnification from the bottom portion of Figure 8-44 shows sclerosing adenosis and acellular fibrous tissue (upper right).

Figure 8-47. Two ducts in continuity contain strikingly different images. The duct on the left is a papilloma, and the one on the right has all the characteristics of ductal adenoma.

Figure 8-44. This sharply circumscribed ductal adenoma has confluent nodules of sclerosing adenosis (bottom), papilloma (lower right), and a densely fibrotic, calcified area.

Figure 8-46. A higher magnification of the right lower portion of Figure 8-44 shows an area indistinguishable from an intraductal papilloma with sclerosis.

Figure 8-48. A higher magnification of Figure 8-47 shows the contiguity of the papilloma and ductal adenoma.

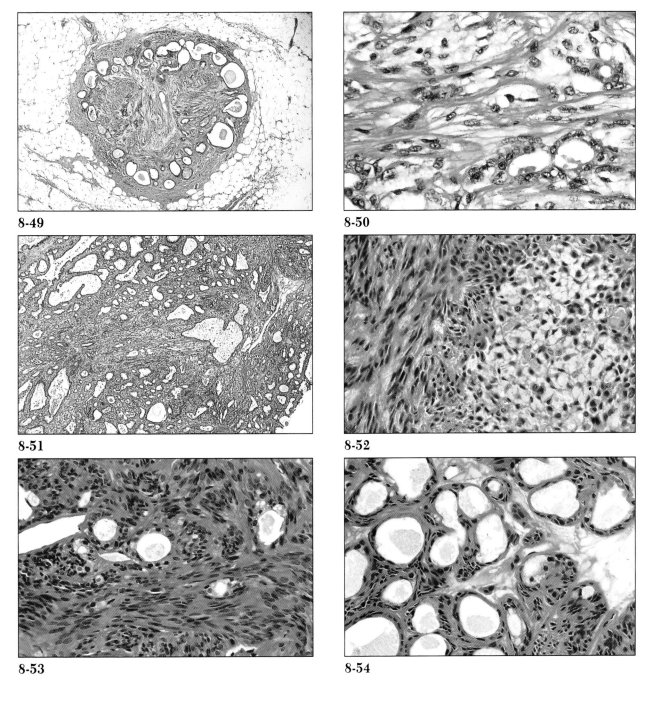

8-49

8-50

8-51

8-52

8-53

8-54

Figure 8-49. This duct has been replaced by a central proliferation of spindled myoepithelial cells and peripheral lumen-forming epithelial cells.

Figure 8-51. Large adenomyoepitheliomas may contain foci of papillary architecture (upper left). Much of this lesion, however, is solid, with a few small lumina and no papillary features.

Figure 8-53. In this example of adenomyoepithelioma, epithelial-lined lumina and fascicles of spindled myoepithelial cells are closely apposed but haphazardly oriented.

Figure 8-50. A higher magnification of Figure 8-49 shows myoepithelial cells with round or elongated nuclei.

Figure 8-52. The spectrum of myoepithelial cells in adenomyoepithelioma includes elongated forms with invisible cell borders, as well as loosely arranged cells with stellate cytoplasm.

Figure 8-54. Some foci of adenomyoepithelioma are composed almost exclusively of glandular elements with only scattered spindled myoepithelial cells.

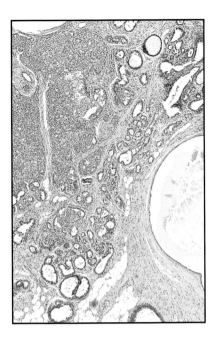

9

PROLIFERATIVE OR ECTATIC PROCESSES OTHER THAN FIBROCYSTIC CHANGE

There are several mammary processes that, although they have some microscopic similarities to fibrocystic change, are best considered as separate entities. Their distinction from typical fibrocystic disease may be based on either clinical or morphologic grounds. One of these conditions, juvenile papillomatosis, is characterized by a clinically detectable mass predominantly composed of marked intraductal epithelial proliferation. At the other extreme is duct ectasia, a nonproliferative process associated with marked duct dilatation.

JUVENILE PAPILLOMATOSIS

Juvenile papillomatosis (so called Swiss-cheese disease of the breast) occurs predominantly in young people. As described below, the individual light microscopic components of juvenile papillomatosis are the same as those discussed in the sections on fibrocystic change. The differences between juvenile papillomatosis and fibrocystic change are predominantly clinical. Juvenile papillomatosis is a discrete, movable mass that does not involve the breast diffusely. The age group of women with juvenile papillomatosis is also far younger than that of women with fibrocystic change. Thus it appears legitimate, based on these features alone, to consider juvenile pap-

illomatosis as a specific entity. Yet another reason for distinguishing juvenile papillomatosis from fibrocystic change relates to the potential role of the former lesion as a risk factor for breast carcinoma in the patient's female relatives.

In the 1985 report by Rosen et al, nine of 180 patients with juvenile papillomatosis had cancer of the breast. Except for a 44-year-old woman with lobular carcinoma in situ in juvenile papillomatosis, all of the women with carcinoma were less than 35 years old. Seven of the women had cancer concurrently with unilateral juvenile papillomatosis. The five ipsilateral synchronous cancers included a 33-year-old woman with multiple foci of lobular carcinoma in situ in the area of juvenile papillomatosis. Another patient, 18 years old, had a secretory carcinoma arising within juvenile papillomatosis. Two women with juvenile papillomatosis had synchronous carcinomas (an infiltrating ductal carcinoma and a secretory carcinoma) in the contralateral breast. Carcinoma of the breast developed asynchronously in two women with bilateral juvenile papillomatosis. One patient had ductal carcinoma in situ, and the other developed a microinvasive ductal carcinoma.

In 1990, Rosen and Kimmel reported the status of 41 women followed up for at least 10 years after the diagnosis of juvenile papillomatosis. Four women developed carcinoma from 5 to 15 years after the initial diagnosis of juvenile papillomatosis. All had a family history of breast cancer. Three of the women were unusual because they had recurrent and bilateral juvenile papillomatosis. The fourth woman had unilateral, recurrent juvenile papillomatosis treated 8 and 12 years before the diagnosis of ductal carcinoma in situ in the contralateral breast. At this writing, none of the women with unilateral but nonrecurrent juvenile papillomatosis had developed carcinoma of the breast.

Patients range from 10 to 44 years of age, but most are 17 to 20 years old. There is nothing unusual about the patterns of menarche, parity, or use of oral contraceptives in these women. There is no reported instance of maternal estrogen therapy administered during pregnancy. Typically, patients have a solitary mass that has been present for a few days to up to 3 years. Sometimes the lesions are multiple, occasionally they are bilateral, and rarely they are a dominant lump in a diffusely nodular breast. Most examples of juvenile papillomatosis are located in the upper outer quadrant, and only a few occur in the subareolar area. On physical examination, the mass is typically firm, circumscribed, and easily movable within the breast. The clinical diagnosis is almost invariably fibroadenoma.

Complete excision of juvenile papillomatosis is effective control for most patients. Nonetheless, 24% of patients with juvenile papillomatosis have undergone subsequent breast biopsies. About two thirds of these have been necessitated by recurrent juvenile papillomatosis. Most of the latter biopsies have been performed in the ipsilateral breast, but about 15% were contralateral. In the absence of juvenile papillomatosis, other changes leading to subsequent biopsy included fibroadenoma, papillomatosis, fibrosis, and mastitis.

Epithelial proliferations in juvenile papillomatosis range from hyperplasia of the usual type to cytologically abnormal hyperplasia coupled with necrosis. The atypical hyperplasia possibly reflects a greater risk of carcinoma analogous to that associated with atypical hyperplasia as a component of fibrocystic changes. However, the long-term risk for patients with juvenile papillomatosis, in general, remains to be determined. Whether subgroups of patients with atypia with or without necrosis are at an increased risk will require study of many more cases and longer follow-up.

Twenty-six percent of patients with juvenile papillomatosis had relatives with carcinoma of the breast. Five of 84 patients had a mother with breast carcinoma and the remaining carcinomas occurred in secondary relatives. It seems likely that relatives of a patient with juvenile papillomatosis are at an increased risk for breast carcinoma, although rigid statistical information to support this contention is still lacking.

On gross inspection, juvenile papillomatosis measures from 1 to 8 cm in greatest dimension. Eighty percent are 5 cm or less in diameter, and one third are less than 3 cm in diameter. The cut surface of juvenile papillomatosis exhibits an irregular, solid nodularity, alternating with cysts 0.1 to nearly 1 cm in diameter. The intervening tissue is fibrous (Figure 9-1).

The diagnosis of juvenile papillomatosis is based on a constellation of individually nonspecific alterations. All cases of juvenile papillomatosis have cysts lined with apocrine, normal, or flattened epithelium (Figure 9-2). In addition, there is papillary apocrine hyperplasia, sclerosing adenosis, duct stasis, and epithelial hyperplasia of the usual type (Figures 9-3, 9-4).

The hyperplasia ranges from mild to florid, and it is indistinguishable from the findings described in the section on fibrocystic changes. Epithelial cells with enlarged and pleomorphic nuclei may be focally present, and 17% of cases are associated with a comedo-type necrosis. The necrosis involves only rare ducts and only a small portion of the affected duct. Exfoliated degenerating cells are also common. Mitotic figures are usually absent but occasionally as many as two or three are seen in ten high-power ($\times$ 400) fields (Figure 9-5). Foamy histiocytes are focally prominent, either in areas of hyperplasia or in nonhyperplastic ducts filled with secretory material (Figure 9-6). Lobules may be discernible and often have an associated proliferation of stroma resembling fibroadenoma. Parenthetically, five of the original 37 patients described by Rosen et al (1980) also had a history of developing fibroadenomas, three of which occurred in the contralateral breast.

DUCT ECTASIA

Duct ectasia involves the larger segmental ducts and collecting ducts, and can result in a palpable tumor. Nipple discharge can occur, and may be serous, bloody, or pasty. Duct ectasia may be accompanied by inflammation and a fibrous reaction, leading to nipple retraction. These symptoms, when accompanied by a palpable mass, almost invariably elicit a clinical diagnosis of carcinoma. Duct ectasia occurs in patients over 30 years of age, with most being between 45 and 70 years of age. At least a mild degree of duct ectasia was seen in half of women older than 60 years of age who had clinically normal breasts at autopsy (Frantz et al).

The pathogenesis of duct ectasia is unknown. A variety of terms have been used, such as *comedomastitis, mastitis obliterans,* and *plasma cell mastitis.* At present, most authors think that these are variants of duct ectasia, and the terms only reflect the variable quantities of inflammation and duct destruction seen in different lesions.

At surgery a cluster of dilated ducts measuring up to 7 mm in size is encountered. The ducts are distended by gray or yellow, grumous material (Figure 9-7). Microscopically, ducts of varying size are closely juxtaposed because of their distension (Figure 9-8). The lumina are filled with amorphous eosinophilic material, and sometimes these contain ovoid crystalline bodies (Figure 9-9). The internal structure of the crystalline bodies is spiculated. Their pathogenesis and composition are unknown. Closely packed crystal-like strands are arranged parallel to one another around the periphery of the body and have a more irregular distribution centrally (Figure 9-10). Rarely, there are intraluminal cholesterol crystals. The lumen may also contain foam cells and, occasionally, multinucleated histiocytes.

The epithelial lining is flattened or absent. Hyperplasia or atypical epithelial changes are not a feature of duct ectasia. An inflammatory response is invariably present. It may consist of a narrow rim of lymphocytes or histiocytes in the duct wall. Sometimes, there is fibrous thickening of the duct wall with only minimal inflammation. In more extreme cases, large numbers of lymphocytes, plasma cells, and histiocytes fill the periductal stroma, and their inflammation is often associated with a marked fibrous response. Ducts may have their epithelial lining replaced by fibrous tissue, including multinucleated histiocytes (Figure 9-11), or the duct lumen may be completely obliterated. An inflammatory infiltrate surrounding the characteristic crystalline bodies described above may be the only remnant of an obliterated duct (Figure 9-12).

REFERENCES

Frantz VK, Pickren JW, Melcher GW, Auchincloss H Jr. Incidence of chronic cystic disease in so-called 'normal breasts.' A study based on 225 postmortem examinations. *Cancer* 1951; 4:762-783.

Haagensen CD. *Diseases of the Breast,* ed 3. WB Saunders Co, Philadelphia, 1986, pp 357-368.

Haagensen CD. Mammary-duct ectasia. A disease that may simulate carcinoma. *Cancer* 1951;4: 749-761.

Kiaer HW, Kiaer WW, Linell F, Jacobsen S. Extreme duct papillomatosis in the juvenile breast. *Acta Pathol Microbiol Scand A* 1979; 87:353-359.

Rosen PP, Cantrell B, Mullen DL, DePalo A. Juvenile papillomatosis (Swiss cheese disease) of the breast. *Am J Surg Pathol* 1980;4:3-12.

Rosen PP, Holmes G, Lesser ML, et al. Juvenile papillomatosis and breast carcinoma. *Cancer* 1985;55:1345-1352.

Rosen PP, Kimmel M. Juvenile papillomatosis of the breast: a follow-up study of 41 patients having biopsies before 1979. *Am J Clin Pathol* 1990;93:599-603.

Rosen PP, Lyngholm B, Kinne DW, Beattie EJ Jr. Juvenile papillomatosis of the breast and family history of breast carcinoma. *Cancer* 1982; 49:2591-2595.

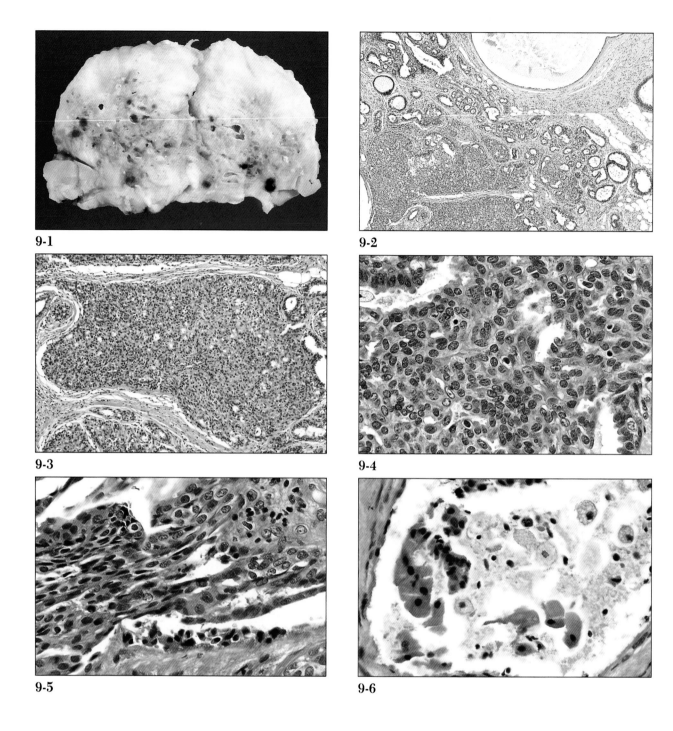

9-1

9-2

9-3

9-4

9-5

9-6

Figure 9-1. The cut surface of juvenile papillomatosis exhibits fibrous tissue, yellow and tan areas of epithelial proliferation, and cysts of varying sizes.

Figure 9-3. The epithelial hyperplasia in this duct of juvenile papillomatosis forms almost solid sheets of cells with only a few lumina.

Figure 9-5. The epithelial component of juvenile papillomatosis may include elongated cells. Degenerating cells are common (bottom).

Figure 9-2. Juvenile papillomatosis typically has elements of epithelial hyperplasia inter-mixed with cysts of varying size. Fibrous tissue surrounds the epithelial elements, as well as extending into surrounding fat.

Figure 9-4. The hyperplasia in juvenile papillomatosis has the angulated spaces and overlapping nuclei characteristics of florid hyperplasia (page 101).

Figure 9-6. Foamy histiocytes are frequently seen in juvenile papillomatosis. In this example, the foam cells are associated with degenerating intraluminal epithelial cells, some of which have apocrine features.

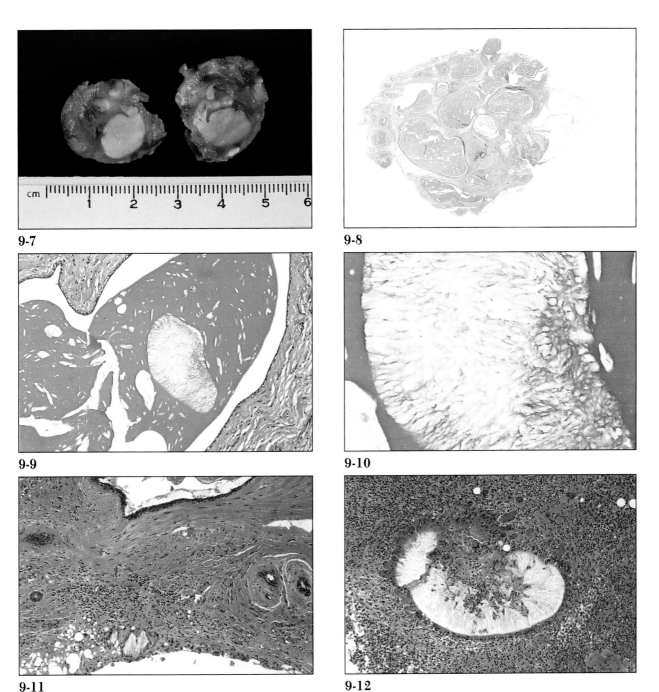

9-7

9-8

9-9

9-10

9-11

9-12

Figure 9-7. Duct ectasia consists of widely dilated ducts containing yellow, tenacious secretions.

Figure 9-9. This cyst of duct ectasia is lined by atrophic epithelium. Dense, eosinophilic secretions are present and these may contain characteristic crystalline bodies, as seen here.

Figure 9-11. The normal epithelial lining of the ectatic ducts may be replaced by histiocytes and foreign body giant cells (bottom).

Figure 9-8. Another example of duct ectasia has cystically dilated ducts filled with secretions. The hyperplastic epithelium of fibrocystic change is not present.

Figure 9-10. The crystalline bodies of duct ectasia have a spiculated internal structure and are of unknown composition.

Figure 9-12. An inflammatory infiltrate with multinucleated histiocytes surrounds a characteristic crystalline body. This may be the only remnant of an obliterated duct in duct ectasia.

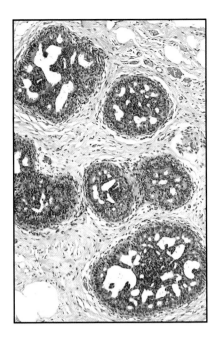

10

UNFOLDING LOBULES AND DUCTAL HYPERPLASIA

A thorough review of the evolution in thinking regarding precancerous lesions of the breast is beyond the scope of this volume. Suffice it to say that studies concerned with precancerous lesions and their site of origin date from the first decades of this century. By the 1920s, hyperplasia was a well-recognized alteration in the breast. In 1931, the "precancerous" potential of some alterations was discussed in detail by Cheatle and Cutler. They and many others thought that lobules and terminal ducts were the initial site of precancerous changes. In 1941, Muir clearly recognized that invasive carcinoma originated from ducts containing what was interpreted as intraductal carcinoma. At approximately this same time, lobular carcinoma in situ was firmly identified.

Current thoughts on the precancerous potential of hyperplasia are also heavily based on a 1945 study by Foote and Stewart, in which nonmalignant portions of carcinomatous breasts were compared with tissue from noncancerous breasts. Hyperplasia, including forms with cytologic atypia, was five times more frequent in the breasts containing cancer.

A number of clinical studies from the 1940s through the 1960s verified an association of "fibrocystic disease" with subsequent carcinoma. These studies recognized that patients who had a biopsy diagnosis of fibrocystic disease were at an increased risk of developing invasive cancer. By the 1970s there were major attempts to separate the histologic components of fibrocystic change in terms of the risk for subsequent cancer.

Before addressing the various components of fibrocystic change, it is necessary to understand the major alterations that the breast can undergo. One must have an understanding of the three-dimensional structure of the elements of fibrocystic change and their relationship to intraductal and in situ neoplasia. To this end, it is critical to visualize the architectural changes resulting from lobular "unfolding." Conventionally, noninvasive proliferations of the breast are viewed as being located in either a lobule or a duct. This terminology is useful for ease in communicating the size of the involved lumen. However, as will be addressed below, many structures that are called ducts actually represent "unfolded" lobules.

Almost all epithelial abnormalities of the breast, including most carcinomas, arise from the terminal duct–lobular unit. This conclusion is based on extensive subgross examinations. With this technique, slices of breast tissue 2 mm thick are prepared by special methods of fixation and sectioning. The word *subgross* refers to the use of a dissecting microscope at a magnification of two to four times. Thus, subgross examination is intermediate between gross and microscopic. Even minimal abnormalities of lobules and their terminal ducts are visible in three dimensions with this technique. After photographing the three-dimensional relationships of a given area, the tissue is embedded in paraffin and stained with H&E for conventional microscopic study. Variations in this approach continue to yield valuable information in conjunction with specimen radiography.

Using the subgross method, Wellings et al proved that the ductules of a lobule can enlarge and the intralobular portion of the terminal duct ceases to be identifiable. The individual ductules usually dilate unevenly, (Figures 10-1, 10-2), and gradually incorporate themselves into a single lumen. The process of ductular enlargement with gradual, progressive effacement of the original lobular architecture is referred to as "unfolding." The lobule remnant eventually is recognizable only by the convoluted outline of one or more lumina (Figure 10-3). Continued dilation of the lobular unit results in spaces the size of small or intermediate segmental ducts (Figure 10-4). Ultimately, the unfolding lobule can eventuate in grossly visible cysts that may be up to a few centimeters in diameter.

At a microscopic level, many of the structures that are designated as subsegmental ducts are derived from the terminal duct–lobular unit after unfolding has taken place. By convention, these structures are referred to as ducts if they have a diameter at least four or five times that of a normal ductule. When these duct-sized structures are close to one another, one can confidently assume that they have arisen from unfolding lobules. Nonetheless, they are called ducts, and they can be the site of hyperplasia or of ductal carcinoma in situ.

Unfolding lobules will sometimes have a serrated border because of the juxtaposition of multiple adjacent ductules that open into a common space. This may result in a papillary appearance (Figures 10-5, 10-6). However, the protrusions of stroma and epithelium lack a delicate fibrovascular core and are thereby distinguished from a true papilloma.

The epithelial cells in unfolding lobules may have elongated nuclei and be more columnar than the epithelium of normal lobules (Figures 10-7, 10-8). The cells may appear stratified when the ductule is cut somewhat tangentially (Figures 10-9, 10-10). This should not be diagnosed as hyperplasia. The epithelium of unfolding lobules, when cut tangentially, may even produce a pseudocrib-

riform pattern (Figures 10-11, 10-12). Unlike cribriform carcinoma (page 112), the cells surrounding the lumina have a "streaming" appearance and are otherwise irregularly distributed. In other lobules, bands of epithelial cells may appear to cross the lumen at apparent points of bifurcation (Figure 10-13) or in areas of luminal irregularity (Figure 10-14). Again, this artifact of sectioning is not to be viewed as hyperplasia. Fortuitous sections through unfolding lobules may occasionally appear as true luminal bridges of epithelium that at low power resemble cribriform ductal carcinoma in situ (Figures 10-15 to 10-18). The cribriform epithelium in unfolding lobules is cytologically normal. It contrasts with the round, sharply demarcated cells with enlarged nuclei characteristic of ductal carcinoma in situ with a cribriform pattern, as illustrated on pages 132 and 133.

Many microscopic, as well as large, cysts of the breast are lined by apocrine epithelium. Apocrine metaplasia begins in the lobule, and it is occasionally seen when the ductules are of normal size or only slightly dilated (Figure 10-19). Progressive unfolding of ductules lined by apocrine epithelium (Figure 10-20) eventually results in lumina that are the size of small ducts. Some of these continue to enlarge to form grossly visible cysts lined by apocrine epithelium. This is the endpoint of unfolded, metaplastic lobules. Ductules or large ducts lined by apocrine epithelium may have papillary infoldings (Figure 10-21). Apocrine epithelium exhibits nuclear pleomorphism, with the largest nuclei ranging from four to six times the diameter of normal nuclei. Nucleoli are often correspondingly enlarged. Nonetheless, there is usually a proportional increase in the volume of cytoplasm, so that the normal nuclear-to-cytoplasmic ratio is maintained (Figure 10-22). Ultrastructurally, the cytoplasm is filled with secretory droplets and a moderate number of mitochondria. This combination produces the granular, eosinophilic cytoplasm seen on H&E-stained sections. Although uncommon, large cytoplasmic vacuoles may be present in apocrine metaplasia, as well (Figure 10-23).

Apocrine epithelium in ducts or cysts frequently forms small tufts and, occasionally, papillae with a central capillary (Figure 10-24). By convention, however, these are not considered to be papillomas. In addition, apocrine epithelium may form looping bridges that are architecturally identical to those seen in usual hyperplasia, atypical hyperplasia, and ductal carcinoma in situ. If the cytologic appearance of the apocrine cells is within the spectrum already described, no special diagnosis is made for these hyperplastic foci.

In their initial study of patients undergoing biopsy for benign breast disease, Page et al (1978) found a slight increase in the risk for cancer in patients with apocrine papillations. This was true, however, only in women beyond the age of 45 years. Their more recent study did not confirm this association. Despite some statements to the contrary (Dixon et al), clinically palpable cysts lined by apocrine epithelium are not currently believed to indicate an increased risk for cancer (Page and Dupont, 1985).

CLINICAL FEATURES OF TYPICAL AND ATYPICAL DUCTAL HYPERPLASIA

Ductal hyperplasia has been accepted as a precancerous lesion for many years. Attempts to quantify ductal hyperplasia in a prognostically relevant fashion were addressed in a 1978 publication by Page et al. These authors studied thousands of benign breast biopsy specimens obtained during the premammographic era from women who had received lengthy clinical follow-up. This database was expanded, and a more detailed analysis of the component parts of "fibrocystic disease" was published in two papers by Page and Dupont in 1985. Recognition of the prognostic relevance of these studies led to a meeting that culminated in the publication of a statement in 1986 entitled "Consensus Meeting: Is 'Fibrocystic Disease' of the Breast Precancerous?" (Hutter). The consensus statement emphasized the differing risks associated with the various microscopic components of ductal epithelial hyperplasia. The majority of women (about 70%) undergoing breast biopsy had little, if any, epithelial hyperplasia. They were not at an increased risk for cancer as compared with the general population. Roughly 25% of women had well-developed hyperplasia and an increased risk for cancer that, when controlled for age, was 1.5 to two times that of the general population.

The risk given in the previous paragraph can also be expressed as the percentage of women who developed invasive carcinoma during the 10- to 20-year follow-up period (median follow-up of 17 years) that was available in their study. Two percent of women with nonproliferative or mildly hyperplastic proliferations developed breast cancer within 15 years, whereas 4% of women with well-developed (moderate or florid) ductal hyperplasia developed breast carcinoma. This is in contrast to the 10% of women who develop breast cancer with atypical ductal hyperplasia (see below).

Atypical ductal hyperplasia is a contentious, "gray zone" diagnosis. The term is applied to ducts having some, but not all, of the architectural and cytologic features of ductal carcinoma in situ. In some ducts, architectural features suggestive of ductal carcinoma in situ will dominate. In others, the architectural features are those of ordinary hyperplasia, but there will be individually atypical cells. Occasionally, features of ductal carcinoma in situ are present, but only involve a small portion of a duct.

If we are to assess risk for subsequent carcinoma, we must apply as carefully as possible the criteria for atypical ductal hyperplasia used by those who have attained follow-up data. The studies of Page and Dupont are the most useful because of their large number of patients with long-term follow-up. It should be emphasized that only 2.1% of specimens representing breast biopsies for benign disease were classified by Page and DuPont as atypical ductal hyperplasia. This term should not be used as a synonym for florid hyperplasia in the absence of architectural or cytologic abnormalities, as this robs it of prognostic meaning. Atypical hyperplasia in the series by Page and Dupont was rarely seen in patients less than 40 years old, but the frequency rose to about 4% in the perimenopausal age group, and it was present in 6% of biopsy specimens from women in their late 60s.

The risk for subsequent invasive carcinoma in patients with either ductal or lobular carcinoma in situ is approximately eight to ten times that of the general population. By comparison, women with atypical ductal hyperplasia are at a moderately increased risk, ie, four to five times that of the general population. Specifically, 18 of 150 women who had atypical ductal hyperplasia developed an invasive breast cancer from 1.4 to 24 years after biopsy. Eight of the 18 women developed carcinoma within 5 years, and 14 had their carcinoma diagnosed within 10 years of biopsy. In ten women (56%) the carcinoma occurred ipsilateral to the atypical ductal hyperplasia. Interestingly, this risk is the same as that for the development of carcinoma in the contralateral breast after mastectomy for invasive

91

carcinoma; namely, 1% of surviving women per year.

PATHOLOGY OF DUCTAL HYPERPLASIA

The usual type of ductal hyperplasia is defined as an increase in epithelial cells, exclusive of apocrine epithelium, small cell lobular-type epithelium, and epithelium with other atypical features. The diverse morphologic patterns of usual (nonatypical) ductal hyperplasia have the common denominator of being populated by benign-appearing cells. The cells have considerable variation in the size, shape, and staining of their nuclei, and quantity of cytoplasm. The majority of nuclei are ovoid, and many round-appearing forms may be short-axis cross sections of ovoid nuclei. The individual nuclei usually have lightly staining chromatin, although considerable chromatic variation is common. Most nuclei are vacuolated, probably reflecting irregular nuclear membranes with many small cytoplasmic invaginations. Nucleoli are usually absent, and, if present, are small and typically single. Mitotic figures are rarely seen, even in florid hyperplasia. Azzopardi, while recognizing that there are no rigid rules for mitotic counts, has stated that a solid epithelial proliferation containing a mitotic figure in every two or three high-power fields is not likely to be benign. This is especially true if abnormal division figures are seen.

The amount of cytoplasm in hyperplastic epithelial cells varies, and it is most often lightly eosinophilic. As with the nuclei, however, there may be considerable difference in the intensity of cytoplasmic staining. Moreover, some cells may have granular cytoplasm closely resembling that seen in apocrine cells. The cell borders are almost always invisible, imparting a syncytial appearance to the epithelium.

The lumen-like spaces seen in hyperplasia are formed passively. They are merely the residua of the original ductal opening that has not been filled with hyperplastic epithelium. This is in contrast to the cribriform variant of ductal carcinoma in situ in which the tumor cells appear to be actively forming lumina (see page 112). In hyperplasia, the arrangement of the cells around lumen-like spaces is variable. Usually, the nuclei are oriented parallel to the opening, a pattern referred to as *streaming*. The streaming layer may be one to several cells thick. The parallel cells may also be arranged in "swirls" or concentric configurations. Although occasionally nuclei appear to be at right angles to a space, the majority are haphazardly oriented. The resultant residual openings vary considerably in size and shape, ranging from narrow slits to larger, irregularly shaped spaces. Only the spaces at the periphery of a duct tend to be more consistently round or slightly ovoid.

The usual type of hyperplasia is subdivided quantitatively into mild, moderate, and florid categories.

Mild hyperplasia is defined as an epithelial layer three or four cells thick. It can occur in ductules, terminal ducts, or large ducts. When mild hyperplasia involves small, slightly dilated ductules, it is difficult to identify the exact thickness of the epithelium because there is often tangential sectioning and apparent bridging (Figures 10-25, 10-26). It is easier to judge the epithelial thickness of widely dilated ductules or ducts, as sections are more likely to transect these structures at approximately right angles. Mild hyperplasia is placed in the category of nonproliferative disease for prognostic purposes. Therefore, the difficulty in interpreting whether or not mild hyperplasia is present is not critical to patient management.

Moderate hyperplasia is an epithelial proliferation that is five or more cells thick. The cells of moderate hyperplasia may be confined to the periphery of the ductule or duct, or form papillae and bridges that cross the ductal lumen (Figure 10-27). The papillae are irregularly shaped and the cells at the tips of the papillae are often smaller than the underlying cells (Figures 10-28, 10-29). More complex proliferations have multiple, "passively" formed spaces at the periphery of the duct (Figure 10-30). Hyperplasia may be confined to only a sector of a duct (Figure 10-31), and may contain cells with apocrine-type cytoplasmic "snouts" (Figure 10-32). Some papillae in hyperplasia may have a "rigid" appearance superficially mimicking micropapillary carcinoma (Figures 10-33, 10-34). However, the overlapping, irregularly shaped nuclei differ from the monomorphic features of micropapillary carcinoma (see page 111). This is not considered an "atypical" pattern. Moderate hyperplasia may have papillae and bridges of epithelium within the same duct (Figures 10-35, 10-36). The epithelial cells lining the longer papillae often have elongated nuclei oriented parallel to the long axis of the papillae (Figure 10-36).

Florid hyperplasia refers to a conspicuous dilatation of ducts with the lumina almost completely filled by epithelial cells (Figures 10-37, 10-38). Moderate and florid hyperplasia are on a continuous spectrum. It is not critical, clinically, to make a sharp distinction between these two grades of hyperplasia, because both are in the same proliferative category for risk assessment of subsequent invasive carcinoma.

The cells of florid hyperplasia often form papillae, but these lack a central capillary, distinguishing them from papillomas (Figures 10-39, 10-40). When these papillae are sectioned transversely, they may appear as "free-floating" cellular islands in the duct (Figure 10-40). The shorter papillae are often club-shaped and have smaller cells at their tips (Figure 10-41). Irregular lumen-like spaces in florid hyperplasia are lined by inconsistently oriented cells (Figure 10-42). Mitotic figures may be present in hyperplasia (Figure 10-42), but these always have a typical configuration.

More extreme examples of florid hyperplasia can almost completely fill involved ducts with the few residual lumen-like spaces typically confined to the periphery (Figure 10-43). In such instances, the most central portion of the proliferation has irregularly distributed nuclei in a "sea" of cytoplasm without discernible cell borders (Figure 10-44). The lumen-like spaces of florid hyperplasia may contain exfoliated, degenerating cells (Figure 10-45). Even in areas with less conspicuous hyperplasia, the luminal cells may assume a shrunken or effete appearance with small, densely hyperchromatic nuclei (Figure 10-46). Solid areas of epithelial hyperplasia are subject to small foci of necrosis in which the cytoplasmic and nuclear debris resembles the necrosis of comedocarcinoma (Figures 10-47, 10-48). The adjacent cells, however, are characteristic of hyperplasia and lack the nuclear atypia of comedocarcinoma.

Some dilated ducts that are almost completely filled with hyperplastic epithelium have more uniformly distributed lumen-like spaces (Figure 10-49). In such cases, close examination will disclose overlapping nuclei and cells unoriented with respect to the lumen-like spaces (Figures 10-50 to 10-52). An even closer mimicry of cribriform carcinoma can occur when florid hyperplasia is composed of cells with more evenly spaced nuclei (Figures 10-53, 10-54). The nuclear variability and overlapping characteristic of typical hyperplasia should predominate, but scattered atypical cells with distinct cell borders may

also be present. When the latter cells are seen in small numbers, the distinction from atypical hyperplasia may be arbitrary (see below) (Figure 10-54).

Florid hyperplasia may have well-formed papillae and bridges of epithelium that mimic micropapillary ductal carcinoma in situ at low magnification (Figure 10-55). The epithelium in these cases, however, lacks the monomorphic appearance of micropapillary ductal carcinoma and, instead, has the overlapping nuclei and irregular cellular arrangement of hyperplasia (Figures 10-56 to 10-58). Lesions such as this that initially evoke a suspicion of ductal carcinoma in situ but lack objective histologic and cytologic criteria should not be interpreted as atypical hyperplasia.

PATHOLOGY OF ATYPICAL HYPERPLASIA

Ductal epithelial proliferations assume a broad range of microscopic appearances. At one end of the spectrum are hyperplasias of the usual type as just discussed. At the other extreme are the various subtypes of ductal carcinoma in situ covered in Chapter 11. Proliferations that have only limited microscopic features of ductal carcinoma in situ are included under the broad term of *atypical ductal hyperplasia*. This designation is used differently by various authors. Before utilizing published risk assessment data, one must be certain that the morphologic criteria applied to a given case are appropriate. In many of the proliferations that we illustrate, our definition of "atypical" hyperplasia differs slightly from that of Page et al, and we have so indicated in the legends.

Atypical hyperplasia has both qualitative and quantitative criteria. The qualitative criteria require a combination of predominantly cytologic abnormalities, in association with an appropriate growth pattern. Having fulfilled the qualitative prerequisites for the diagnosis of atypia, atypia can be graded as mild to severe, based in great part on the quantity of the abnormalities. For example, a rare, well-formed lumen fully typical of cribriform ductal carcinoma in situ can occur in a duct otherwise involved with hyperplasia. Because the quantity of the abnormal cells and their abnormal architecture is minimal, this can be viewed as mild atypia. Conversely, if most of the duct is involved, it can be viewed as severe atypia.

The diagnosis of atypical hyperplasia can be made when there is partial involvement of a duct by alterations architecturally and cytologically indistinguishable from cribriform carcinoma. For example, lumen-like spaces may be focally lined by cells with basally oriented nuclei and discrete cell borders, as is typical of cribriform carcinoma (Figures 10-59 to 10-62). Architectural abnormalities resembling micropapillary carcinoma occur when bridges and papillae are formed at the periphery of a duct (Figure 10-63). The streaming of cells and the ovoid, overlapping nuclei distinguish these lesions from carcinoma or atypical hyperplasia (Figures 10-64, 10-65). However, when such foci contain scattered, cytologically atypical cells they may be labeled as atypical hyperplasia (Figure 10-66).

Cytologic atypia may be present in association with any degree of epithelial hyperplasia, but is more common in the moderate to florid forms. In our experience, cytologic atypia most commonly consists of individual cells with enlarged nuclei and distinct cell borders interspersed in an otherwise typical focus of hyperplasia (Figures 10-67, 10-68). This phenomenon of isolated atypical cells has not been emphasized, and the associated risk for invasive carcinoma has not been addressed in the literature.

Cytologically abnormal cells may also form aggregates or sheets that partially involve a duct (Figures 10-69, 10-70). Because there is only partial ductal involvement, an unequivocal diagnosis of ductal carcinoma in situ is not warranted. Instead, a diagnosis of atypical hyperplasia is appropriate. As with single-cell atypia, the risk assessment for ducts partially involved with these larger aggregates of variably atypical cells is difficult to discern.

Finally, atypical hyperplasia may lack a specific architectural arrangement but consist of numerous cytologically abnormal cells with high nuclear to cytoplasmic ratios, irregular shapes, and hyperchromatic nuclei (Figures 10-71, 10-72). If some or many of the cells in the duct are still characteristic of usual-type hyperplasia, the diagnosis of atypical hyperplasia is made.

REFERENCES

Azzopardi JG. *Problems in Breast Pathology.* WB Saunders Co, Philadelphia, 1979, p 121.

Cheatle GL, Cutler M. *Tumours of the Breast. Their Pathology, Symptoms, Diagnosis and Treatment.* JB Lippincott, Philadelphia, 1931, p 161.

Dixon JM, Lumsden AB, Millard WR. The relationship of cyst type to risk factors for breast cancer and the subsequent development of breast cancer in patients with breast cystic disease. *Eur J Cancer Clin Oncol* 1985;21:1047-1050.

DuPont WD, Page DL. Risk factors for breast cancer in women with proliferative breast disease. *N Engl J Med* 1985;312:146-151.

DuPont WD, Page DL. Relative risk of breast cancer varies with time since diagnosis of atypical hyperplasia. *Hum Pathol* 1989;20:723-725.

Foote FW, Stewart FW. Comparative studies of cancerous versus noncancerous breasts. *Ann Surg* 1945;121:6-53,197-222.

Hutter RVP. Consensus meeting. Is 'fibrocystic disease' of the breast precancerous? *Arch Pathol Lab Med* 1986;110:171-173.

Muir R. The evolution of carcinoma of the mamma. *J Pathol Bacteriol* 1941;52:155-172.

Page DL. Cancer risk assessment in benign breast biopsies. *Hum Pathol* 1986;52:155-172.

Page DL, DuPont WD. Are breast cysts a premalignant marker? *Eur J Cancer Clin Oncol* 1985;21:635-636.

Page DL, DuPont WD, Rogers LW, Rados MS. Atypical hyperplastic lesions of the female breast. A long-term follow-up study. *Cancer* 1985;55:2698-2708.

Page DL, VanderZwaag R, Rogers LW, et al. Relation between component parts of fibrocystic disease complex and breast cancer. *JNCI* 1978;61:1055-1063.

Tesluk H, Amott T, Goodnight JE Jr. Apocrine adenoma of the breast. *Arch Pathol Lab Med* 1986;110:351-352.

Tham K-T, Dupont WD, Page DL, et al. Micropapillary hyperplasia with atypical features in female breasts, resembling gynecomastia. *Prog Surg Pathol* 1989;10:101-109.

Wellings SR, Jensen HM, Marcum RG. An atlas of subgross pathology of the breast with special reference to possible precancerous lesions. *JNCI* 1975;55:231-273.

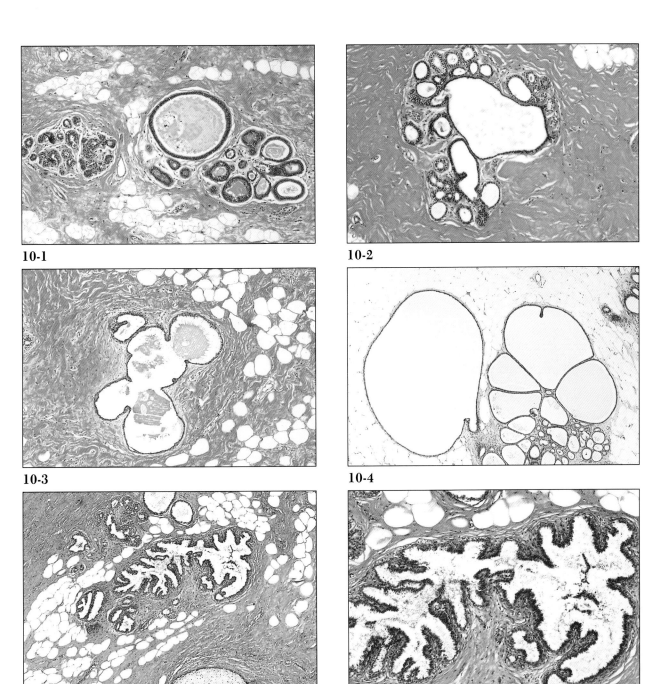

10-1

10-2

10-3

10-4

10-5

10-6

Figure 10-1. A normal lobule is present at left. At right, the individual ductules of an unfolding lobule dilate unevenly.

Figure 10-3. The convoluted outline of several fused ductules helps distinguish this unfolded lobule from a subsegmental duct.

Figure 10-5. Unfolding lobules may have a serrated border created by the fusion of adjacent ductules. This image should not be confused with a papilloma.

Figure 10-2. Dilating ductules gradually become confluent, creating larger lumina equal in size to small ducts.

Figure 10-4. Dilation of a lobular unit may create spaces the size of large subsegmental ducts.

Figure 10-6. A higher magnification of Figure 10-5 confirms the lack of capillaries in the papilloma-like protrusions of an unfolding lobule.

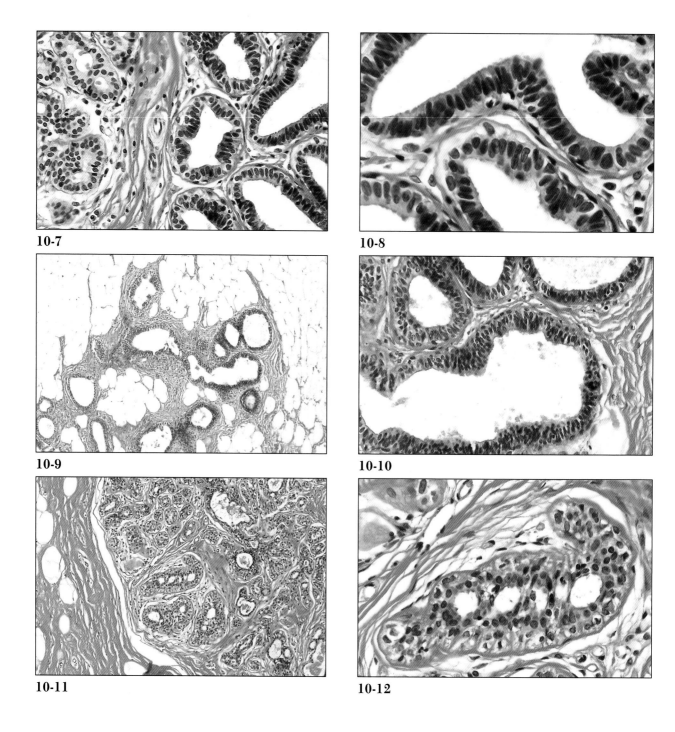

10-7

10-8

10-9

10-10

10-11

10-12

Figure 10-7. As compared with the normal lobule on the left, the unfolding lobule on the right has slightly larger lumina. The epithelial cells of the unfolding lobule have larger, elongated nuclei.

Figure 10-9. The elongated cells in an unfolded lobule may become stratified as the ductules progressively dilate. When the ductules are separated by fat, as seen here, the process has been termed "blunt duct adenosis."

Figure 10-11. Small ductules beginning to unfold, when sectioned tangentially, may have a cribriform-like appearance (center).

Figure 10-8. The epithelial cells of this unfolding lobule are columnar.

Figure 10-10. The epithelial cells in unfolding lobules may have stratified nuclei. Where the epithelium is cut at approximately right angles, it is two cells thick. Tangential sectioning produces areas of greater apparent thickness, but this should not be considered hyperplasia.

Figure 10-12. A higher magnification of Figure 10-11 shows that streaming epithelium separates the apparent lumina. The irregularly distributed nuclei also distinguish this artifact from cribriform carcinoma (page 112).

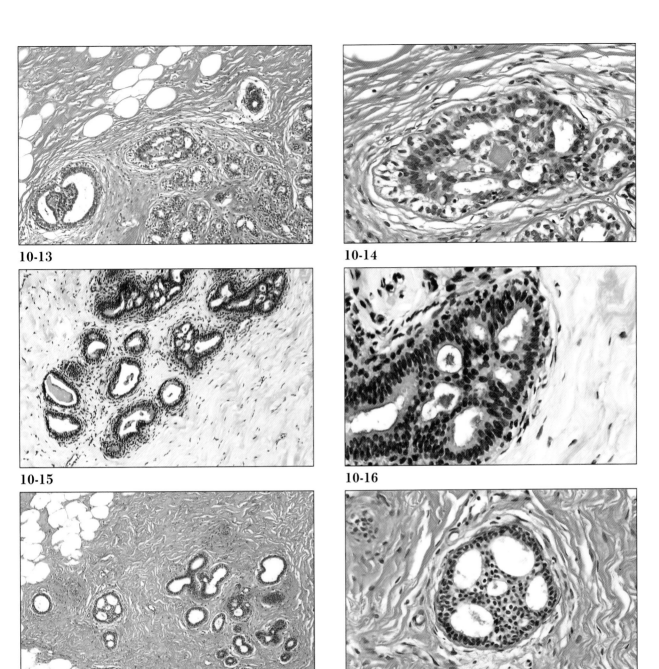

10-13

10-14

10-15

10-16

10-17

10-18

Figure 10-13. Fortuitous sections through unfolding ductules can create seemingly complex epithelial patterns. The ductule at left is interpreted as a section at a point of bifurcation.

Figure 10-15. Fortuitous sections through unfolding lobules may also mimic cribriform carcinoma. This is a common occurrence in ductules of this size.

Figure 10-17. The ductule with several lumina at left resembles cribriform carcinoma at low power.

Figure 10-14. A higher magnification of another ductule from Figure 10-13 shows multiple, irregularly shaped lumina. The apparent complexity created by the plane of section should not be diagnosed as hyperplasia.

Figure 10-16. A higher magnification from Figure 10-15 shows a cribriform-like ductule. The cells at the periphery of the ductule retain their orientation with basal nuclei. However, the more central cells are randomly distributed with respect to the lumen-like spaces.

Figure 10-18. A higher magnification of Figure 10-17 shows more even nuclear distribution than in Figures 10-15 and 10-16. However, there is sufficient variation in the cells to exclude the monomorphism of cribriform carcinoma (page 112).

98

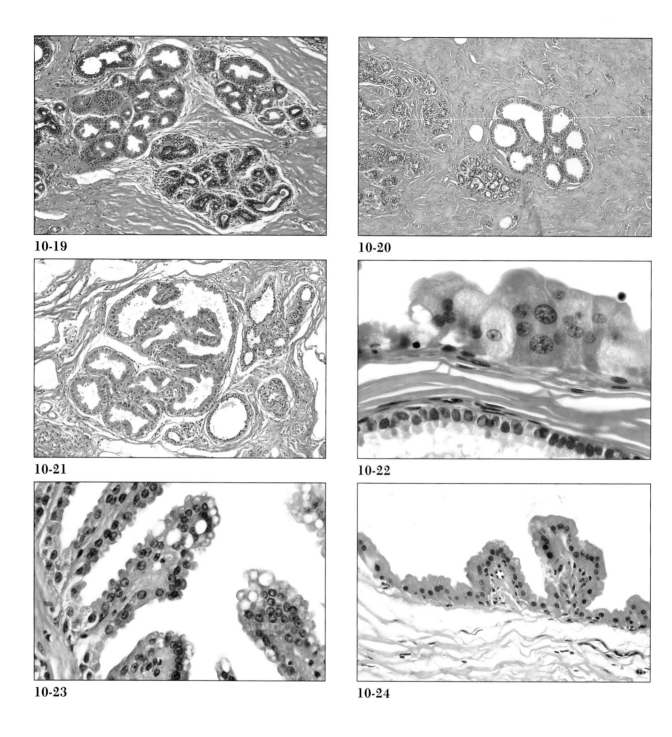

10-19

10-20

10-21

10-22

10-23

10-24

Figure 10-19. Apocrine metaplasia begins in the lobule and is occasionally seen when only minor lobular unfolding is present.

Figure 10-21. As the apocrine-lined ductules become even more widely dilated, they may acquire irregular papillary infoldings.

Figure 10-23. Large cytoplasmic vacuoles, as seen here, are uncommonly encountered in apocrine metaplasia.

Figure 10-20. In this example of apocrine metaplasia, the ductules are markedly dilated when compared with the adjacent lobule. Nonetheless, their close apposition confirms their lobular origin.

Figure 10-22. This example of apocrine epithelium exhibits marked nuclear pleomorphism. The largest nuclei are four to six times the diameter of the normal nuclei in the adjacent duct.

Figure 10-24. Apocrine epithelium in ducts or cysts frequently forms small tufts and, occasionally, papillae with a central capillary may be seen. Despite the presence of central capillaries, these are not conventionally considered to be papillomas.

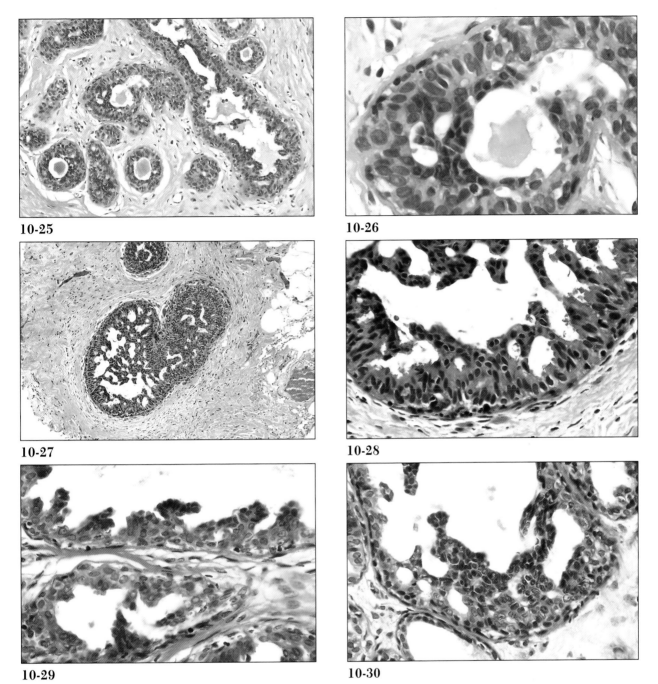

10-25

10-26

10-27

10-28

10-29

10-30

Figure 10-25. Mild hyperplasia, as seen here, is defined as an epithelial layer three or four cells thick. In slightly dilated ductules of this size, the epithelial bridges are probably due to tangential sectioning and should not be used as a criterion for moderate or florid hyperplasia.

Figure 10-27. Moderate hyperplasia, as seen here, is an epithelial proliferation more than five cells thick. The epithelium can form bridges across the lumen or papillae.

Figure 10-29. The irregularly shaped papillae in this example of moderate hyperplasia have bland, overlapping nuclei.

Figure 10-26. The innermost layer of hyperplasia has smaller cells. These cells also compose the artifactual bridges.

Figure 10-28. The thickened epithelium of moderate hyperplasia often forms papillae. The cells at the tips of papillae are frequently small with dense nuclei.

Figure 10-30. This more complex variant of moderate hyperplasia has multiple "passively" formed spaces at the periphery of the duct.

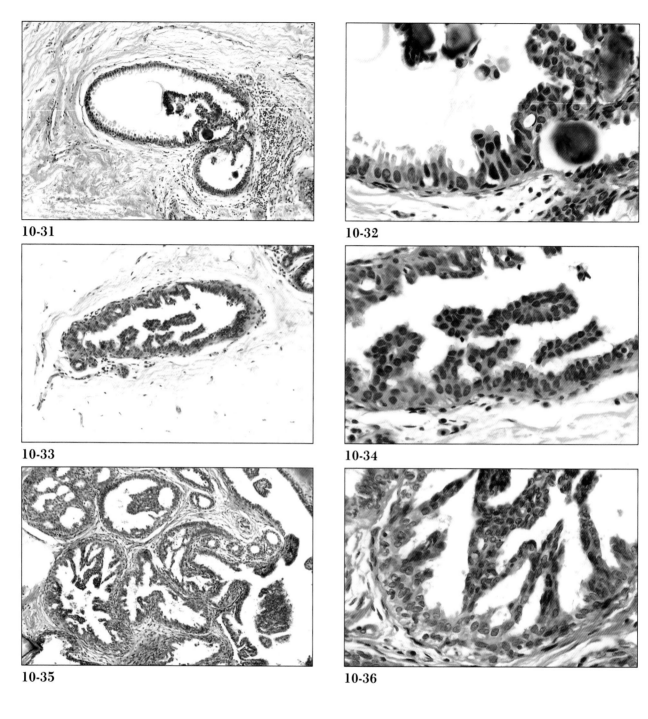

10-31

10-32

10-33

10-34

10-35

10-36

Figure 10-31. Hyperplasia may involve only one sector of a duct. Foci of calcification, as seen here, may also be present.

Figure 10-33. These papillations in moderate hyperplasia enter the lumen at right angles and have a "rigid" appearance.

Figure 10-35. This example of moderate hyperplasia has architecturally variable papillary proliferations.

Figure 10-32. This higher magnification of Figure 10-31 shows variably shaped, overlapping nuclei. Note the apocrine epithelium at the left, as well as the multiple micro-calcifications.

Figure 10-34. A higher magnification of Figure 10-33 shows overlapping, irregularly shaped nuclei, lacking the monomorphic features of micropapillary carcinoma (page 111).

Figure 10-36. The epithelial cells lining the right-angle papillations in hyperplasia often have elongated nuclei oriented along the axis of the papilla.

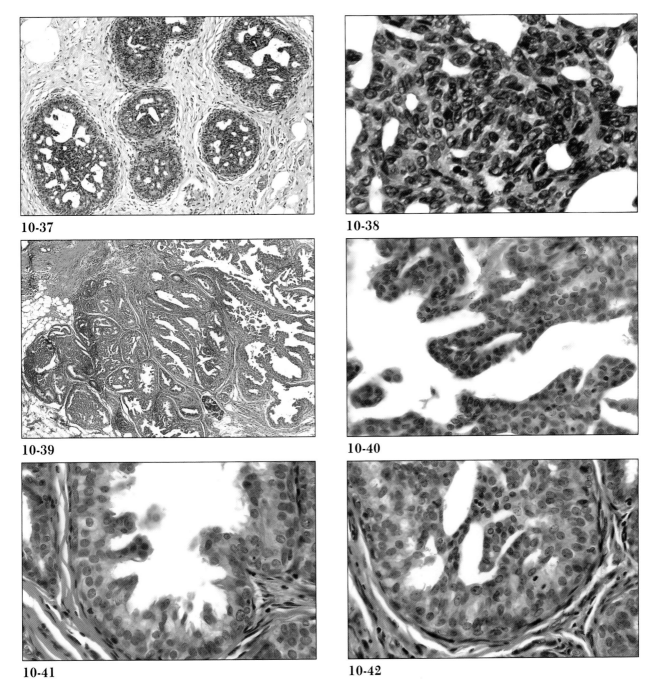

10-37

10-38

10-39

10-40

10-41

10-42

Figure 10-37. In florid hyperplasia, most of the lumen is replaced by epithelium, leaving irregular, often angulated spaces.

Figure 10-39. The epithelial proliferation of florid hyperplasia fills most of the duct lumen.

Figure 10-41. Right-angle papillae often have smaller and denser nuclei at their tips. The papillae are frequently club-shaped.

Figure 10-38. A higher magnification of Figure 10-37 discloses overlapping nuclei and irregular arrangement of cells around the residual luminal spaces.

Figure 10-40. The papillae of florid hyperplasia lack a fibrovascular core, distinguishing them from papillomas.

Figure 10-42. Irregular, lumen-like spaces in florid hyperplasia are lined by inconsistently oriented cells. Mitotic figures, as seen here, may be present in hyperplasia, but these always have a typical configuration.

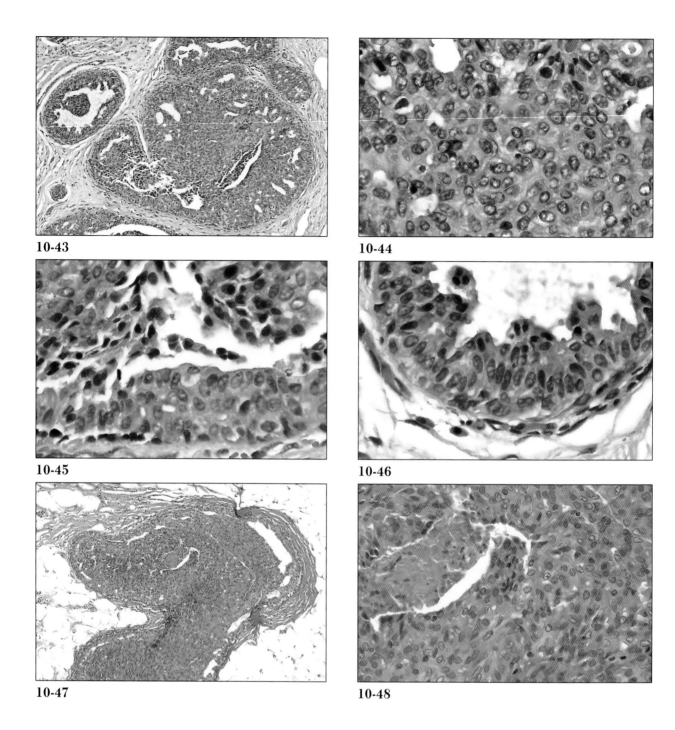

10-43

10-44

10-45

10-46

10-47

10-48

Figure 10-43. Florid hyperplasia may be an almost completely solid epithelial proliferation filling the duct. The lumen-like spaces that remain are concentrated at the periphery.

Figure 10-45. Another higher magnification of Figure 10-43 shows that the luminal epithelial cells are exfoliated as they degenerate. This should not be confused with comedocarcinoma.

Figure 10-47. Hyperplastic epithelium completely fills the duct, except for peripheral irregular spaces. A small area of necrosis is present.

Figure 10-44. The central portion of the epithelial proliferation seen in Figure 10-43 has irregularly distributed nuclei, resulting in small islands of cytoplasm without discernible cell borders.

Figure 10-46. A higher magnification of Figure 10-43 shows that the cells of the deeper layers have plump, "active" nuclei. The more superficial cells have small, contracted nuclei and less cytoplasm.

Figure 10-48. A higher magnification of Figure 10-47 shows that the necrosis is associated with cells having the typical nuclear variability of hyperplasia.

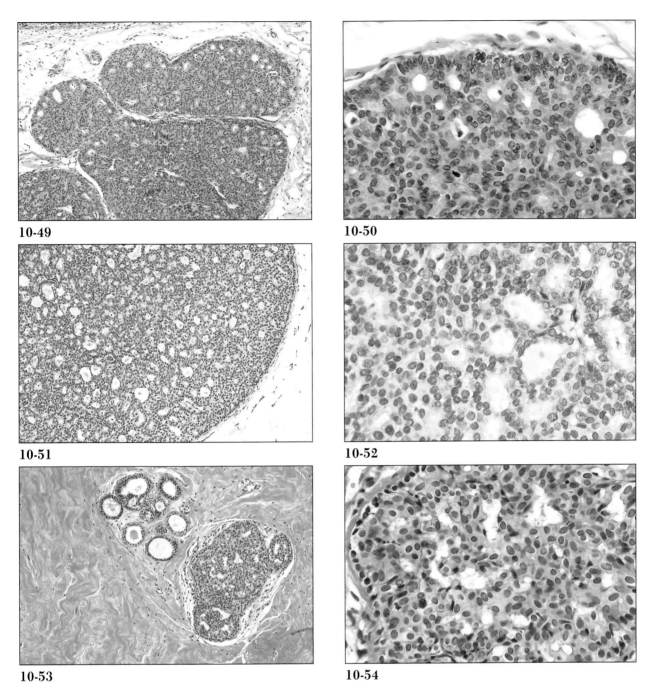

10-49

10-50

10-51

10-52

10-53

10-54

Figure 10-49. These dilated ducts are almost completely filled with hyperplastic epithelium.

Figure 10-51. This large duct has numerous lumen-like spaces resembling cribriform ductal carcinoma in situ at low magnification.

Figure 10-53. Florid hyperplasia with irregular lumen-like spaces has more evenly spaced cells than are seen in Figure 10-51.

Figure 10-50. A higher magnification of Figure 10-49 shows ovoid, overlapping nuclei that are irregularly distributed. In addition, they are unoriented with respect to the lumen-like spaces.

Figure 10-52. A higher magnification of Figure 10-51 illustrates the bland, variably sized nuclei of ductal hyperplasia. The epithelial cells have no constant orientation with respect to the lumen-like spaces.

Figure 10-54. A higher magnification of Figure 10-53 shows that the more evenly spaced cells nonetheless have the nuclear variability characteristic of hyperplasia. Compared with Figure 10-51, a larger number of cells have well-defined cell borders. Some would consider this to be hyperplasia with cytologic atypia, but the predominant pattern is typical.

UNFOLDING LOBULES AND DUCTAL HYPERPLASIA

104

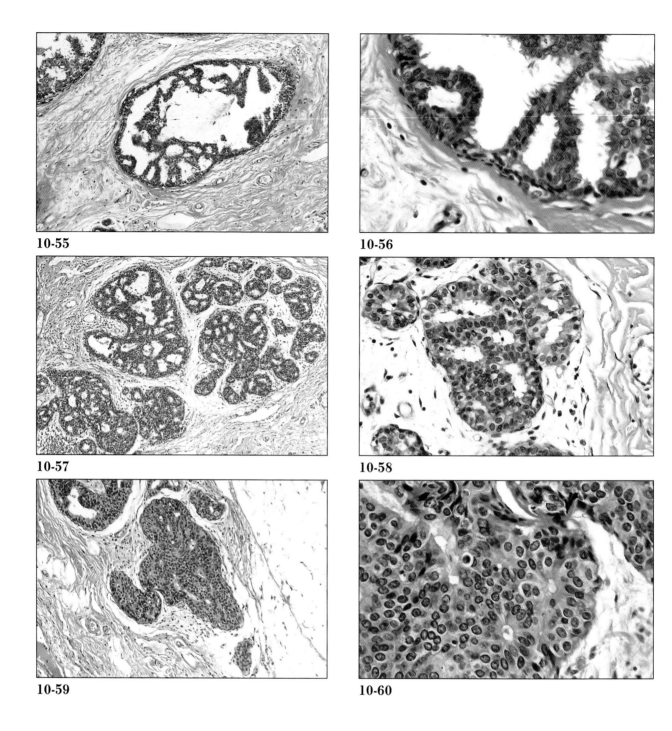

10-55

10-56

10-57

10-58

10-59

10-60

Figure 10-55. Ductal hyperplasia may form papillae and bridges that mimic micropapillary ductal carcinoma in situ.

Figure 10-57. This example of florid hyperplasia has numerous bridges of epithelium, resulting in irregularly shaped lumina that mimic a mixture of cribriform and micropapillary carcinoma.

Figure 10-59. This example of atypical hyperplasia has cells completely filling the duct lumen.

Figure 10-56. A higher magnification of Figure 10-55 shows that the "Roman bridges" of epithelium have ovoid, overlapping nuclei characteristic of hyperplasia. The apocrine "snouts" seen here are of no value for distinguishing hyperplasia from carcinoma.

Figure 10-58. A higher magnification of Figure 10-57 again demonstrates the overlapping nuclei and lack of cell orientation around lumen-like spaces that typify ductal hyperplasia.

Figure 10-60. Higher magnification of Figure 10-59 discloses a small opening near the bottom of the field, suggesting true lumen formation of cribriform ductal carcinoma in situ. A few cells have sharply defined cell borders at lower right. These features warrant the diagnosis of atypical hyperplasia.

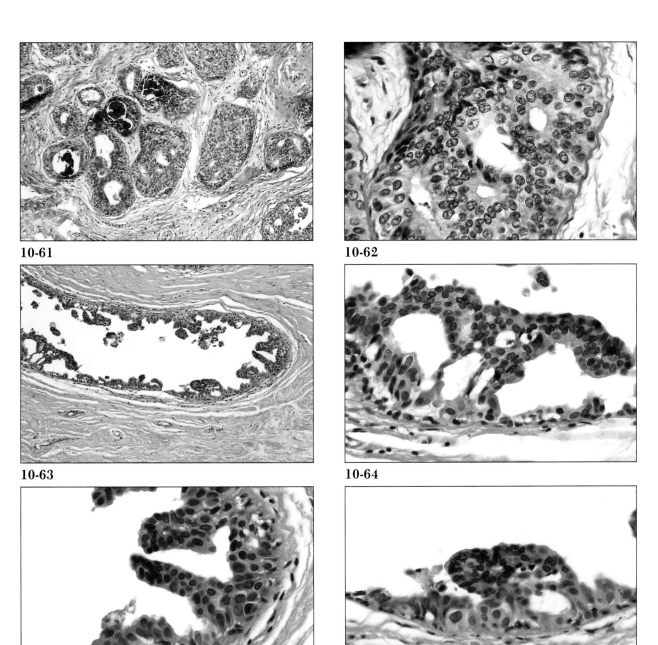

10-61

10-62

10-63

10-64

10-65

10-66

Figure 10-61. At low magnification, this example of atypical hyperplasia has ducts that display the spectrum of appearances seen in usual florid hyperplasia, including irregular lumen-like spaces and almost completely filled ducts. The microcalcifications are of no diagnostic value.

Figure 10-63. Florid epithelial hyperplasia of the usual type may form bridges and papillae resembling micropapillary ductal carcinoma in situ at low magnification.

Figure 10-65. Another higher magnification of Figure 10-63 discloses papillae with irregularly arranged cells and cytologic variation typical of hyperplasia.

Figure 10-62. A higher magnification of Figure 10-61 shows that most cells have overlapping and ovoid nuclei characteristic of usual hyperplasia. Streaming of the hyperplastic cells is prominent at the lower right. However, two lumina are lined by cells with basally oriented nuclei. This orientation is identical to that of cribriform carcinoma. We interpret this field as an example of atypical hyperplasia.

Figure 10-64. A higher magnification of Figure 10-63 shows the ovoid, overlapping nuclei and cell "streaming" of hyperplasia.

Figure 10-66. A few cells from Figure 10-63 have increased amounts of powdery cytoplasm and enlarged nuclei. Cells of this type, when they form a monomorphic population, are characteristic of cribriform and micropapillary ductal carcinoma in situ.

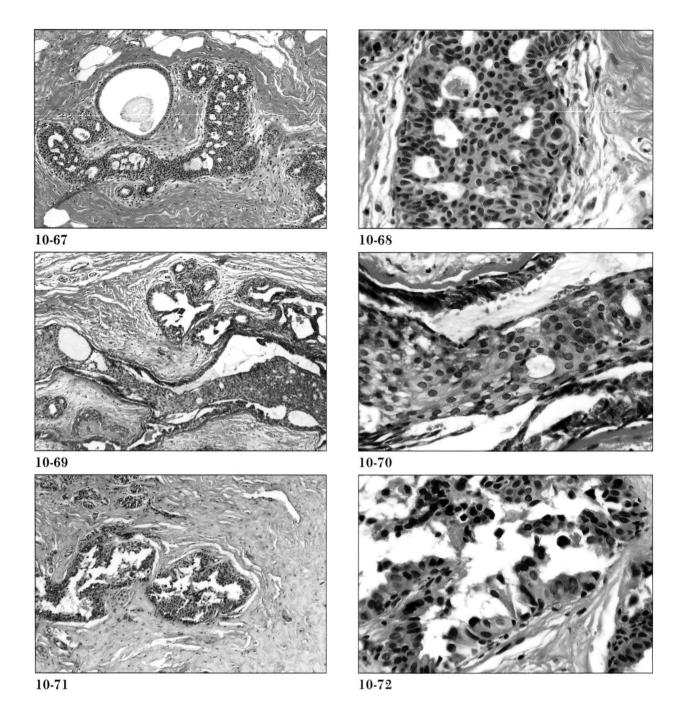

10-67

10-68

10-69

10-70

10-71

10-72

Figure 10-67. This atypical intraductal proliferation has the appearance at low magnification of florid hyperplasia of the usual type.

Figure 10-69. A duct with atypical hyperplasia contains a long, almost solid strand of monomorphic cells mixed with the characteristic cells of hyperplasia.

Figure 10-71. This example of atypical hyperplasia has numerous cytologically abnormal cells.

Figure 10-68. A higher magnification of Figure 10-67 shows irregular lumen-like spaces characteristic of hyperplasia. However, occasional large nuclei are seen in cells with sharply defined cell borders. We interpret this as atypical hyperplasia on the basis of these focal cytologic abnormalities.

Figure 10-70. A higher magnification of Figure 10-69 shows an island of predominantly monomorphic cells traversing the lumen. The monomorphic cells have powdery, eosinophilic cytoplasm and evenly spaced nuclei.

Figure 10-72. A higher magnification of Figure 10-71 shows cells with high nuclear-to-cytoplasmic ratios. The nuclei are irregular in shape and many are hyperchromatic. Other areas of the duct, such as at lower left, are lined by cells of usual-type hyperplasia.

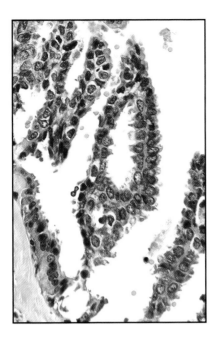

11

DUCTAL CARCINOMA IN SITU

In the early 1900s, it was suggested that there were morphologically recognizable preinvasive lesions of the breast, and this concept was crystallized in Broders' paper on carcinoma in situ, published in 1932. He defined carcinoma in situ as "a condition in which malignant epithelial cells and their progeny are found in or near positions occupied by their ancestors before the ancestors underwent malignant transformation. At least they have not migrated beyond the juncture of the epithelium and connective tissue or the so-called basement membrane." Specifically relevant to carcinoma in situ of the breast, he stated: "In adenocarcinoma in situ the malignant cells often completely replace the nonmalignant cells in what were once normal acini, ducts, or tubules." It is self-evident that invasive carcinomas of the breast arise from transformed epithelium that originates within ducts or lobules. Moreover, these transformed cells must, for some period of time, be noninvasive. Several observations validate the concept of carcinoma in situ. These include the cytologic identity of many invasive cancers with their intraductal counterparts, microscopic foci of continuity between intraductal lesions and invasive carcinomas, and epidemiologic studies demonstrating an increased risk for subsequent invasive carcinoma in women with ductal carcinoma in situ treated only with local excision.

CLINICAL ASPECTS

In the premammographic era, ductal carcinoma in situ presented in one of three ways. It may have been an incidental microscopic finding, usually consisting of only a few ducts, in a biopsy of a clinically suspicious, palpable mass. The patient almost always had multiple palpable abnormalities, and the excised mass, the so-called "dominant lump," usually had fibrocystic changes. The second manner of presentation was as a palpable mass that resulted from a large number of closely packed carcinomatous ducts. Finally, some patients presented with bleeding or discharge from the nipple (Schuh et al, Millis and Thynne). Women with nipple discharge or bleeding sometimes have diffuse but nonpalpable ductal carcinoma in situ (Andersen et al, 1988). These presentations of ductal carcinoma obviously still occur. To them, however, has been added mammographically worrisome abnormalities that are nonpalpable and asymptomatic.

It is possible that the biologic behavior of ductal carcinoma in situ in these three clinical groups is different, even for a given subtype of in situ carcinoma (Patchefsky et al, 1989) (Gump et al). The quantity of ductal carcinoma in situ varies tremendously in these situations. This is most conspicuous when comparing the incidentally found ductal carcinoma in situ (as in the setting defined above) and the quantity of ductal carcinoma in situ that results in a palpable mass. The quantity of mammographically detected nonpalpable ductal carcinoma in situ usually falls between these extremes. Nonetheless, many mammographically identified, nonpalpable breast cancers are multicentric, which is defined as involvement of quadrants other than that containing the primary lesion. In the study by Schwartz et al (1980), nine of 18 cases of ductal carcinoma in situ were multicentric.

The clinical relevance of subclassifying ductal carcinoma in situ is becoming progressively refined. It is particularly important to separate comedocarcinoma from other forms of ductal carcinoma in situ. When compared with nonnecrotic types of ductal carcinoma in situ, comedocarcinoma has the highest rate of concomitant invasion at the time of first diagnosis. Lacking initial invasion, comedocarcinoma has a higher likelihood of subsequent invasive carcinoma if untreated. There is a greater probability that the invasive carcinoma will be cytologically identical to the comedocarcinoma. Cell kinetic studies demonstrate a higher labelling index in comedocarcinoma, as compared with nonnecrotic ductal carcinoma in situ (Meyer). Micropapillary ductal carcinoma in situ also has a proclivity for microinvasion (30%), as well as a high rate of multicentricity when compared with other types of ductal carcinoma in situ. By contrast, the cribriform and solid types of intraductal carcinoma tend to have fewer involved ducts and a low frequency of multicentricity. These two variants of ductal carcinoma in situ exhibited no microinvasion in the series by Patchefsky and associates (1989).

Until recently, there were only a few reported patients with intraductal carcinomas of various types treated by biopsy alone. Rosen et al (1980) reviewed the literature and identified eight patients with comedocarcinoma that were otherwise untreated. Six (75%) developed invasive carcinoma in less than 4 years.

Page et al reported 28 women with micropapillary ductal carcinoma in situ who had been treated by biopsy alone. Of the 22 patients who were followed up for 3 years or more, seven (32%) developed an ipsilateral invasive carcinoma. It should be noted that two of the original 28 patients had concomitant lobular carcinoma in situ. Whether this independently increased the risk is currently unanswerable. The study by Betsill et al reported on 25 women with cribriform or micropapillary ductal carcinoma in situ who were not treated further. Only 15 women were available for follow-up, including ten with long-term follow-up averaging 22 years. In seven of the ten patients, ipsilateral invasive cancer developed at a mean interval of 9.7 years. In addition to ductal carcinoma in situ, two women had lobular carcinoma in situ in the initial biopsy specimen. It is difficult to use this series for risk assessment because of the many patients without follow-up. Eusebi et al followed up 28 patients with ductal carcinoma in situ for a minimum of 16 years. Three developed ipsilateral invasive carcinoma from 5 to 12 years after the original biopsy.

Webber et al followed up women with ductal carcinoma in situ treated with mastectomy and found no increase in invasive cancer in the contralateral breast. Autopsy studies have shown a high frequency of contralateral ductal carcinoma in situ in women with invasive carcinoma, which implies that not all foci of ductal carcinoma in situ become invasive.

The studies by Lagios and associates on all types of ductal carcinoma in situ are especially illuminating. Their group has been treating women with a small volume of ductal carcinoma in situ by local excision (tylectomy). In an earlier study, they examined 53 mastectomy specimens after a biopsy diagnosis of ductal carcinoma in situ (type not further specified). The specimens were studied by the serial subgross sectioning technique that maximizes the detection of ductal carcinoma in situ and clinically occult invasive cancers. Not unexpectedly, this method more frequently detects occult invasion than simply taking random samples from all quadrants of a mastectomy. The authors found that 21% of their patients had occult invasive carcinomas. Ductal carcinoma in situ was considered to be multicentric if another focus was found 50 mm or farther from the reference tumor. None of the 29 cases of ductal carcinoma in situ measuring 25 mm or less had occult invasive carcinoma in the mastectomy, although four had multicentric foci and two had involvement of the nipple. By contrast, 11 of 24 lesions that were 26 mm or greater in size had occult invasion and 13 were multicentric. Thus, it seemed reasonable to treat ductal carcinoma in situ by local excision when it was less than 25 mm in size. Other clinical considerations must be taken into account, however, such as ease of breast examination and the presence of a family history of breast cancer.

Thus far, Lagios and colleagues (1989) have followed up 79 women after tylectomy. The cases have been divided into four histologic subtypes using a combination of cytologic and architectural features. Type I is typical comedocarcinoma characterized cytologically by cells with large, markedly atypical nuclei. Architecturally, the cells form solid sheets. Type II has cytologically identical cells, but they are distributed in an irregular papillary or cribriform pattern, resulting in lumen formation. Type III consists of smaller, less pleomorphic cells than Types I and II. Necrosis, if present, appears only in punctate foci. Type IV is defined as ductal carcinoma in situ with small, uniform cells forming either cribriform and/or micropapillary patterns. Necrosis is absent. Mixed forms of ductal carcinoma in situ are categorized according to the ducts that have the highest grade of nuclear abnormality, even if they constitute a minority of the tumor (Lagios, personal communication, 1989).

Eight (10%) of the 79 women in the series by Lagios and colleagues (1989) have developed a recurrence of either ductal carcinoma in situ or invasive carcinoma. All recurrences have been ipsilateral. Five (16%) of 31 women with Type I comedocarcinomas treated with tylectomy have had a recurrence and two (40%) of five women with Type II ductal carcinoma in situ have had recurrence. One (10%) of the ten women with Type III carcinoma had a recurrence. Most importantly, none of the 33 women with Type IV ductal carcinoma in situ has had recurrent disease thus far.

Similar recommendations for conservative therapy have been made by Patchefsky et al (1989) for ductal carcinoma in situ incidentally found by breast biopsy performed for benign disease. As mentioned earlier, the number of ducts involved in this clinical situation is usually few, and in Patchefsky and colleagues' (1989) study of subsequent mastectomies, there was no additional ductal carcinoma in situ.

There is little information regarding a purported rare variant of micropapillary ductal carcinoma in situ that has been called *cystic hypersecretory duct carcinoma.* Partial excision of hypersecretory ductal carcinoma in situ has been followed by persistent enlargement, although no such case has as yet eventuated in an invasive carcinoma. Interestingly, four of 29 patients with hypersecretory ductal carcinoma in situ had invasive cancer at the time of the initial diagnosis (Guerry et al). The invasive carcinomas were not adjacent to the hypersecretory in situ lesions, however, and the infiltrating components were high-grade tumors with minimal evidence of secretory activity or lumen formation. It has been suggested that hypersecretory ductal carcinoma in situ is better viewed as an unusual hypersecretory form of hyperplasia (Jensen and Page).

MICROSCOPIC FEATURES

As stated in the introduction, the most reproducible intraductal lesions associated with the highest risk for invasive carcinoma are called ductal carcinoma in situ or its interchangeable term, intraductal carcinoma. The former designation is used in this volume because it parallels the well-established term lobular carcinoma in situ. There is no widely accepted classification for the conspicuously different cytologic and architectural arrangements that are included under the rubric of ductal carcinoma in situ. Nonetheless, five broad patterns of ductal carcinoma in situ can be identified: comedocarcinoma, micropapillary, cribriform, solid, and papillary. Approximately one third of patients with ductal carcinoma in situ have two or more of the patterns to be described (Patchefsky et al, 1989). Not surprisingly, the greater the number of ducts involved, the greater the chance that different patterns will be seen.

Cytologically, some lesions display a continuum in cell size from the smallest cells of micropapillary or cribriform ductal carcinoma in situ to the largest cells of comedocarcinoma. The architectural arrangements likewise overlap. For example, an otherwise typical, large cell comedocarcinoma may have well-formed lumina, imparting a cribriform-like appearance. Conversely, tumors with abundant central necrosis may consist of small, uniform cells, as seen in cribriform or micropapillary carcinomas, and maintain a well-formed cribriform or micropapillary architecture in the intact cells. There are no specific rules for classifying these tumors with mixed patterns. Patchefsky et al (1989) classified mixed lesions based on the dominant histologic pattern, which generally consisted of 60% to 70% of the tumor, and, as discussed above, Lagios et al (1989) classify such lesions according to the highest nuclear grade.

110

Before illustrating the several types of ductal carcinoma in situ, two points are in order regarding semantics. As stated previously, Wellings et al have demonstrated that most breast lesions, including ductal carcinoma in situ, arise from the terminal duct–lobular unit. Clear evidence for this can be found in many cases of ductal carcinoma in situ when one's attention is directed to the lobules rather than to the most conspicuously enlarged ducts. The lobules may have cytologic or architectural changes, or a combination of alterations that are identical to those in the large ducts containing ductal carcinoma in situ. Often, there is the distinct impression that the abnormalities are arising in the lobule and are not a secondary extension from the duct (Figures 11-1 to 11-6). The most definite evidence for the lobular origin of many ductal carcinomas is found when lobules contain both cytologic and architectural features typical of ductal carcinoma in situ (Figures 11-7 to 11-10). Even when ductules have been enlarged to the point where they are the size of subsegmental ducts, the large number of such ducts per unit area is indicative of their origin from the many ductules of a single lobule (Figures 11-11, 11-12).

Micropapillary ductal carcinoma in situ and cribriform ductal carcinoma in situ are often characterized as having a monomorphic population of cells. It is important to understand the concept of a monomorphic population because it is commonly used as one criterion for the diagnosis of some forms of ductal carcinoma in situ, as well as lobular carcinoma in situ. What constitutes a monomorphic population is subjective, and it does not mean that every cell is identical. The cytoplasm in different cells can have the same tinctorial quality, but the quantity may vary greatly. Some cells may have apocrine snouts. In such instances, one nonetheless has the impression that the cells are qualitatively monomorphic, despite the variable volumes of cytoplasm. Similarly, nuclei in a monomorphic population can differ in size and shape. Even if nuclei were perfectly spherical and of identical size, there would be variation in their diameter in histologic preparations because of differences in the plane of section. Moreover, even a small deviation from a perfect sphere compounds this variation. Most micropapillary and cribriform carcinomas have at least a few cells with ovoid nuclei, and often they are numerous. As with the quality of the cytoplasm, if the quality of the nuclear staining is approximately the same, and the

variation in size and shape is minimal, one may conclude that the nuclei are those of a monomorphic population. It should be emphasized that the presence of a preserved myoepithelial layer is not evidence against a monomorphic population. Most examples of ductal carcinoma in situ replace the normal epithelial and myoepithelial lining, but in many instances the myoepithelial layer is partly or completely preserved. Its presence is not a criterion against the diagnosis of ductal carcinoma in situ.

A small proportion of cells in ductal carcinoma in situ may only loosely fit the definition of a monomorphic population. These cells may be physically distorted by compression or stretching so that their nuclei are markedly elongated. The cytoplasm of the cells may be so attenuated that it is difficult to assess its quality. Although it may be impossible to objectively recognize these cells as a part of a monomorphic neoplastic population, as long as they are not clearly distinct, they can be interpreted as consistent with the otherwise monomorphic neoplasm.

Illustrations of the ductal carcinoma in situ prototypes included in this monograph can serve as a source for comparison with less diagnostic images encountered in practice. Depending on the features of the less characteristic ducts, they may be interpreted as variants of ductal carcinoma in situ or, if they lack sufficient features, diagnosed as atypical ductal hyperplasia.

Comedocarcinoma

The quantity of necrosis in ductal carcinoma in situ usually, but not always, reflects the cytologic constitution. The greater the number of necrotic ducts, the greater the chance that the tumor is composed of large, cytologically high-grade cells. Approximately 85% of in situ ductal carcinomas with necrosis are of high nuclear grade (Patchefsky et al, 1989). By definition, necrosis, unless in rare microscopic foci, excludes the category of solid ductal carcinoma in situ. Necrosis is uncommon in micropapillary and cribriform carcinomas composed of small cells. Therefore, it is quite reasonable to make necrosis the overriding criterion for the classification of comedocarcinoma.

Comedocarcinoma is the form of intraductal carcinoma that most often presents as a palpable mass and is the easiest to suspect on gross examination. The large ducts with their necrotic debris are easily recognizable grossly, and the necrotic material can be expressed with slight pressure (Figure 11-13). Microscopically, comedocarcinoma typically consists of a thickened layer of cells at the periphery of a duct surrounding a central mass of necrotic, granular, cytoplasmic debris, intermixed with nuclear fragments. The cells around the periphery may be irregularly distributed with true lumina (Figure 11-14), or solid sheets of cells (Figure 11-15).

The cells of comedocarcinoma exhibit a broad spectrum of cytologic appearances. They may be rather uniform and only slightly larger than normal (Figure 11-14). Alternately, they may be markedly enlarged and clearly abnormal with a high nuclear-to-cytoplasmic ratio (Figure 11-16). The cytoplasm may be predominantly clear (Figure 11-16), but more often is eosinophilic (Figure 11-17). The luminal layer of epithelium is often flattened and slightly retracted from the necrotic debris (Figure 11-18). This distinguishes the necrosis typical of comedocarcinoma from that seen in juvenile papillomatosis, nipple adenomas, and hyperplasia of the usual type. In these benign conditions, the intact epithelial cells most often blend with the necrotic cells and remain in continuity with them. Clearly, however, the latter pattern may also be encountered in comedocarcinoma (Figure 11-16). When the cells of comedocarcinoma are cytologically bland and show some "streaming" or compression, they may be difficult to recognize on purely cytologic grounds. Nonetheless, the presence of a central lumen filled with necrotic debris should strongly raise the possibility of comedocarcinoma (Figures 11-19 to 11-22). This suspicion is heightened if there are remnants of normal epithelium at the edge of a duct containing abnormal cells (Figure 11-21, right side). Two other helpful features for distinguishing cytologically bland comedocarcinoma from hyperplasia are the typically tight compression of comedocarcinoma cells, and the often flattened inner (luminal) layer, as described above.

Comedocarcinoma may also exhibit considerable architectural variation. Foci of seemingly complex epithelial proliferation may be due to the involvement of closely apposed ductules, as well as larger ducts (Figures 11-23, 11-24). Still other examples may display a combination of micropapillary and cribriform patterns. In such instances, the cells may be evenly spaced, form rigid bridges, and have the abundant powdery cytoplasm that characterizes many intraductal micropapillary or cribriform carcinomas (Figures 11-25, 11-26). More complex papillary structures may arise in comedocarcinoma (Figures 11-27, 11-28). Whether these are interpreted as comedocarcinoma or micropapillary/cribriform ductal carcinoma in situ with necrosis is arbitrary. Ducts containing comedocarcinoma may be lined by only one or two neoplastic cells, and necrosis may focally denude the lining (Figures 11-29 to 11-34). The presence of only a thin layer of neoplastic cells has been referred to as "clinging carcinoma" (Eusebi et al).

Rarely, the initial microscopic manifestation of comedocarcinoma is "embolized" intraductal necrosis or necrotic debris associated with exfoliated atypical cells in otherwise benign ducts (Figures 11-35, 11-36). The presence of intraluminal necrotic debris should always stimulate extensive sectioning of the tissue block in order to substantiate the diagnosis of carcinoma by finding intact, malignant cells.

Micropapillary Carcinoma

This variant of ductal carcinoma in situ sometimes presents as a mass (Figure 11-37) because of the aggregation of innumerable dilated ducts (Figure 11-38). Unlike comedocarcinoma, necrotic debris cannot be expressed, and the tumor has a firm consistency.

Micropapillary ductal carcinoma has a highly variable microscopic appearance. The term reflects the fact that tumor cells form small broad, narrow, or branching papillations that are roughly at right angles to the duct wall (Figure 11-39). By definition, the papillations are devoid of fibrovascular cores, distinguishing the lesion microscopically from intraductal papillary carcinoma. In addition, the cells may form looping arches (Roman bridges) and complex spoked-wheel or arcade arrangements (Figure 11-40). The vertical papillae frequently have a "rigid" appearance (Figure 11-41).

Micropapillary ductal carcinoma in situ may have elongated cells, some of which appear to be "streaming." The cells at the tips of papillae are often smaller than those at the bases (Figures 11-41, 11-42). Small, effete cells are also commonly seen lining the tips of papillae in usual hyperplasia. In both instances, this change may reflect a physiologic process in which the cells at the greatest distance from the underlying vascular supply have become "nutritionally deprived." Regardless of the mechanisms involved, the fact that the papillae of micropapillary ductal carcinoma in situ may have smaller cells centrally does not detract from the concept of a monomorphic population. Sometimes, the well-preserved peripheral neoplastic cells of micropapillary ductal carcinoma in situ impart a "pseudopagetoid" appearance (Figures 11-43, 11-44). This probably represents the same phenomenon in which the more central cells become smaller, with denser cytoplasm and contracted nuclei (Figure 11-44).

The quantity and configuration of the epithelium in a given duct containing micropapillary carcinoma in situ can vary considerably. Occasionally, the ducts are filled and expanded with complex proliferations to the point of being visible grossly (Figure 11-45). Microscopically, the neoplastic epithelium may form complex intersecting bridges (Figures 11-46 to 11-48), or be concentrated mainly at the periphery of the duct (Figures 11-49, 11-50). Only a sector of a duct may be involved (Figures 11-51 to 11-54), often with an abrupt junction between normal and neoplastic epithelium (Figure 11-52). Partially involved ducts provide an excellent opportunity to contrast the cytologic features of the normal and neoplastic cells. The partial involvement of ducts may be accompanied by a mixture of solid as well as papillary patterns (Figure 11-55). The involved ducts may retain a layer of normal cells that merges with the neoplasm (Figure 11-56). Some of the epithelial bridges may be partially involved with neoplastic cells, with other, smaller cells being indistinguishable from usual hyperplasia (Figure 11-57). Similarly, the more solid proliferations may feature a mixture of neoplastic and apparently hyperplastic cells (Figure 11-58).

Micropapillary ductal carcinoma in situ usually consists of a monomorphic population of small cells. However, some architecturally atypical examples are composed of intermediate to large cells with vesicular nuclei and a modest degree of pleomorphism (Figures 11-59 to 11-62). Some epithelium resembles apocrine epithelium (Figures 11-63, 11-64). Other cells have scant cytoplasm (Figures 11-65, 11-66). Ducts involved with micropapillary ductal carcinoma in situ also may consist of moderately large cells with well-defined cell borders, accompanied by small uniform cells with minimal cytoplasm (Figures 11-67, 11-68). This raises the possibility that some ductal carcinomas in situ are composed of multiple monomorphic populations. This hypothesis would account for ducts that have abnormal cells differing in size or configuration (Figures 11-69, 11-70).

Ductal carcinoma in situ may almost completely fill the lumen, leaving irregular spaces resembling those of hyperplasia. This can be viewed as a case of extensive involvement with micropapillary ductal carcinoma in situ or incomplete involvement with solid ductal carcinoma in situ (Figures 11-71, 11-72). The presence of conspicuous secretory material or cytoplasmic debris within the lumina should heighten the concern that a proliferation represents ductal carcinoma in situ rather than hyperplasia.

Intracytoplasmic lumina are rarely seen in ductal carcinoma in situ, whereas they are common in lobular carcinoma in situ (see page 150). If the lumina lack a dense droplet of secretory material, they have the appearance of signet-ring cells. When a central aggregate of dense secretions is seen in an intracytoplasmic lumen, the cell is often referred to as a "target cell" (Figures 11-73, 11-74). As with lobular lesions, the presence of target and signet-ring cells in ductal proliferations increases the likelihood that the lesion is carcinoma. Rarely, micropapillary carcinoma in situ confined to the periphery of the duct may have small areas of necrosis. Again, it may be arbitrary whether such proliferations are considered unusual variants of comedocarcinoma or micropapillary carcinoma with focal necrosis (Figures 11-75, 11-76). If a monomorphic population of small cells is present, this argues more strongly for the interpretation of micropapillary carcinoma with focal necrosis.

Rosen and Scott have described what they consider to be a variant of micropapillary ductal carcinoma in situ in which a large number of closely approximated, dilated ducts are present (Figures 11-77, 11-78). Many ducts have dense luminal secretions, and Rosen and Scott propose the term *cystic hypersecretory carcinoma* for this lesion. The ducts may be partially or totally lined by short papillae of small to moderate-sized cells. Some have slightly vacuolated cytoplasm, suggesting active secretion.

Cribriform Carcinoma

The third type of ductal carcinoma in situ consists of ducts that are partly or completely filled with neoplastic cells forming lumina. The lumina may be of variable size, but usually are round, rather than forming the irregularly shaped openings of ordinary hyperplasia. In its most well-developed form, the luminal cells of cribriform carcinoma are low columnar, evenly spaced, and radially oriented with the nuclei in the basal portion of the cytoplasm (Figures 11-79, 11-80). In other instances, the lumina are lined by a layer of round or low cuboidal cells (Figures 11-81, 11-82). Interluminal secretions may be prominent, and associated with calcification (Figures 11-81, 11-82).

The lobular origin of cribriform ductal carcinoma in situ is occasionally obvious when the involved ducts are small and have a lobular configuration or are associated with ductules containing cytologically identical cells (Figures 11-83, 11-84).

The ducts of cribriform carcinoma may be greatly enlarged, resembling ductal adenoma at low power (Figure 11-85). At higher magnification, however, the well-oriented periluminal cells are apparent (Figure 11-86). Occasionally, the lumina are irregularly shaped and formed by cells with a less clearcut orientation, such that at low power they resemble hyperplasia (Figures 11-87, 11-88). When ductal carcinoma in situ forms many variably shaped lumina, some of which are separated by only a few neoplastic cells, the diagnosis of cribriform vs micropapillary ductal carcinoma in situ becomes arbitrary (Figures 11-89 to 11-92).

Some intraductal epithelial proliferations have focal, round, lumen-like spaces, but lack a monomorphic cell population (Figures 11-93 to 11-96). In such foci, cells may be radially oriented around the lumen as in cribriform ductal carcinoma in-situ, and these foci can be considered architecturally atypical. However, in the absence of a monomorphic population, the diagnosis of ductal carcinoma in situ is untenable, and such foci are better interpreted as atypical ductal hyperplasia.

Cribriform ductal carcinoma is mimicked by collagenous spherulosis (Figures 11-97, 11-98). This term was coined by Clement et al for ducts having intraluminal clusters of eosinophilic spherules. The spherules are surrounded by round to oval epithelial cells with scant cytoplasm and bland nuclei. The epithelial component of collagenous spherulosis is identical to that of ordinary ductal hyperplasia. Type IV collagen composes part of the spherules, indicating that they contain a component of basement membrane material (Clement et al).

Cribriform intraductal carcinoma also must be distinguished from adenoid cystic carcinoma of the breast (Figures 11-99 to 11-102). Round, widely separated islands of invasive adenoid cystic carcinoma can resemble multiple cribriform ducts or micropapillary carcinoma. The basal-like cells are cytologically distinctive and are unlike the round cells of cribriform carcinoma. The cells of adenoid cystic carcinoma are not oriented with respect to the lumen-like spaces, and the cells often have overlapping nuclei.

Solid Carcinoma

In this variant, ducts are partially or completely filled with neoplastic cells lacking a specific pattern (Figure 11-103). Rarely, a remnant of normal or hyperplastic ductal cells can be seen along the edges of the neoplastic component (Figure 11-104). Some examples of solid carcinoma have microscopic necrosis (Figure 11-104), but more than rare foci of necrosis in a ductal carcinoma in situ should lead to the diagnosis of comedocarcinoma. The cytologic appearance ranges from cells with moderate amounts of partially clear cytoplasm (Figures 11-103, 11-104) to cells with powdery cytoplasm (Figures 11-105, 11-106). Solid ductal carcinoma in situ need not fill the entire duct (Figures 11-107, 11-108, 11-111, 11-112). On occasion, the cytologically abnormal cells are loosely cohesive, with foci of degeneration (Figures 11-109, 11-110). Other forms of solid ductal carcinoma in situ will have a low-power pattern suggestive of hyperplasia with preservation of irregular lumina (Figure 11-111). In all these variations, higher magnification should demonstrate that the cells are sufficiently pleomorphic and atypical to clearly justify the diagnosis of ductal carcinoma in situ (Figure 11-112).

Occasional ducts are populated by variably atypical cells, many of which are unrecognizable as clearly malignant (Figures 11-113, 11-114). This is especially true when the cells resemble apocrine epithelium by having pleomorphic nuclei and granular, eosinophilic cytoplasm. Ducts completely filled with such cells are highly suggestive of carcinoma in situ (Figures 11-115, 11-116). Ducts that are not completely filled with such epithelium are less worrisome, although they may represent an earlier stage of evolution to solid ductal carcinoma in situ (Figures 11-117, 11-118). Intraductal epithelial proliferations such as this serve as reminders that many proliferative lesions undoubtedly represent ductal carcinoma in situ, but are unrecognizable as such unless accompanied by a cytologically identical infiltrating component (Figures 11-119, 11-120).

Papillary Carcinoma

In this variant, the epithelium lines branching, fibrovascular stalks. A fibrovascular core does not occur in any of the other forms of ductal carcinoma in situ. The unifying feature of a fibrovascular papillary stroma in papillary ductal carcinoma in situ encompasses a number of cytologic and histologic variations. The cells are often stratified, and oriented perpendicular to the connective tissue stalks (Figures 11-121, 11-122). Cytoplasm may be conspicuous or, more commonly, it is sparse, or barely discernible. Nuclei might be lightly (Figure 11-122) or densely stained (Figures 11-123, 11-124), or vesicular with irregular chromatin clumping (Figures 11-125, 11-126). The cytologic spectrum includes both the small, uniform cells typical of micropapillary or cribriform ductal carcinoma and larger, more pleomorphic cells similar to those of solid ductal carcinoma or comedocarcinoma.

Papillary ductal carcinoma in situ can assume any of the patterns seen in other forms of ductal carcinoma in situ by superimposing these configurations on a fibrovascular stalk. For example, there may be Roman bridges, tufts, or secondary papillary protrusions devoid of a capillary (Figures 11-127 to 11-130). Epithelial proliferations can bridge the spaces between fibrovascular stalks, creating irregularly shaped lumina (Figures 11-131, 11-132). Solid sheets of epithelial cells may also be present. The nonpapillary lining of a duct containing papillary carcinoma may have the same abnormal cell population as the papillary component, or it may be lined by normal epithelium.

MICROINVASION

A biopsy specimen containing predominately lobular or ductal carcinoma in situ plus grossly undetectable areas of invasion suggests that the patient is at risk for metastasis, and therefore indicates the presence of life-threatening disease. The risk for metastasis is difficult to assess because of differing termi-

nology and criteria regarding what constitutes microinvasion or minimally invasive carcinoma. In many instances, one or more easily recognized microscopic foci of invasive carcinoma are seen. Tumor cells that are irregularly scattered in fat or are situated in fibrous tissue between ducts or lobules pose no problem in diagnosis. Indeed, some studies have quantitated the percentage of invasive tumor as compared with ductal carcinoma in situ. The ratio of invasive carcinoma to carcinoma in situ has been shown to have prognostic significance when the invasive element makes up a small percentage of the lesion (Patchefsky et al, 1977; Silverberg and Chitale).

A more difficult problem revolves around the interpretation of minute foci of questionable microinvasion. The latter term is used with the recognition that it has no widely accepted definition. For the purposes of this discussion, we define microinvasion as nests of cells immediately adjacent to ducts showing ductal carcinoma in situ. Utilizing this definition, microinvasion cannot extend more than 0.1 mm from the duct. Similar criteria could be applied to lobular carcinoma in situ but, in fact, the question of microinvasion, as we have defined it, rarely arises in association with this lesion.

We agree with Page and Anderson that the "overdiagnosis of focal invasion has frequently been the standard of practice in the past." The tendency for overdiagnosis stems from the irregular contour of ducts containing carcinoma in situ and involvement of contiguous ducts and lobules. In the latter situation, the individual ductules are often sectioned in a plane that does not confirm the continuity of the lobule with the carcinomatous duct.

Seemingly discontinuous nests of atypical epithelial cells can usually be distinguished from invasive carcinoma by evaluating several microscopic criteria. A smooth outer contour of the cell nests favors ductular extension, whereas an irregular contour suggests microinvasion. When irregular epithelial nests are accompanied by a looser fibrous reaction than is present elsewhere around the duct, this is substantiating evidence for invasion. Occasionally, normal epithelial cells will remain in the protrusions of epithelium, confirming their noninvasive character (Figures 11-133, 11-134). In other instances, the collagen around the epithelium has a laminated appearance that follows the contour of the protruding epithelium (Figures 11-135, 11-136). Even when epithelial nests have markedly irregular contours, sharply defined and closely apposed collagen should discourage their interpretation as microinvasion (Figures 11-137, 11-138). Experimental studies have suggested that invasion may be heralded by defects of basement membrane immunoperoxidase components such as collagen type IV and laminin, as identified by immunoperoxidase stains (Charpin et al). The diagnostic utility of these techniques requires further study, however.

When the epithelial-stromal junction is blurred, it may be arbitrary as to whether or not this is interpreted as the earliest manifestation of invasion (Figures 11-139, 11-140). The problem is heightened when the population of protruding cells is slightly different cytologically from the clearly intraductal component (Figures 11-141, 11-142). Unequivocal evidence of microinvasion consists of irregularly shaped and variably sized nests of cells surrounded by a "fresh" fibroblastic proliferation that is not well oriented around the individual epithelial nests (Figures 11-143, 11-144).

If a prominent lymphocytic infiltrate is adjacent to the suspicious epithelium and is more abundant than the lymphocytes around the ductal carcinoma in situ, this further supports a diagnosis of microinvasion. In fact, a dense lymphocytic aggregate should always be inspected closely for tumor cells, even if there is no ductal carcinoma in situ on the remainder of the slide. The study by Haupt et al is pertinent to this observation. These authors examined breast tissue from patients with axillary lymph node metastases and no clinically detected carcinoma in the breast. In the women who underwent mastectomy, the subsequently detected infiltrating carcinoma often had a prominent lymphocytic infiltrate, even in the absence of grossly visible tumor. In several cases, the lymphoid infiltrate was the first microscopic clue to the presence of carcinoma, although it sometimes required step sections to find the neoplastic cells.

Different microscopic forms of intraductal carcinoma are associated with different frequencies of microinvasion. Patchefsky et al (1989) found that, overall, 29% of their patients with ductal carcinoma in situ had microinvasion. Almost all of those patients with invasion had comedocarcinoma as their in situ lesion. However, Patchefsky et al also found microinvasion in three of ten micropapillary tumors, whereas none of the solid or cribriform variants of ductal carcinoma in situ had invasion. Although there was no direct relationship with the number of ducts involved, there was a tendency for invasion to occur in cases with larger volumes of ductal carcinoma in situ. Nevertheless, the authors emphasized that there was no minimal number of involved ducts that precluded invasion.

Even in the absence of demonstrable invasion, about 1% of patients with ductal carcinoma in situ, lobular carcinoma in situ, or both will have positive axillary lymph nodes (Rosen et al, 1980). Such cases presumably represent unavoidable sampling errors or, perhaps, involuted foci of invasion. Origin from ectopic breast tissue is a remote possibility (Walker and Fechner). Whatever the reason, it is clear that extensive sectioning will occasionally fail to identify invasion, even in patients with positive lymph nodes. This is exemplified by one reported case in which the patient had two positive axillary lymph nodes, but 180 sections from the tumor biopsy specimen failed to show invasion (Patchefsky et al, 1989).

UNUSUAL VARIANTS OF DUCTAL CARCINOMA IN SITU

Intracystic Carcinoma

Intracystic carcinoma is a somewhat vague term that has been applied by some to a heterogenous group of sharply demarcated, cystlike carcinomas. We believe that it should be more appropriately reserved for ductal carcinoma in situ, usually of papillary type, that involves a dilated, grossly visible duct (Figure 11-145). Carter et al classified papillary ductal carcinoma in situ as intracystic carcinoma when the involved duct measured more than 1 cm in diameter. Intracystic carcinomas up to 14 cm in greatest dimension have been reported. Regardless of size, however, this is a noninvasive carcinoma that does not metastasize. Nevertheless, Carter et al emphasized that it is imperative to closely examine the small ducts outside the intracystic component. If ductal carcinoma in situ of any type is present outside the intracystic component, there is an increased risk for development of invasive carcinoma.

Intracystic carcinoma may be predominantly solid on gross examination if the duct is filled with neoplastic cells. More often, there is a greatly dilated cyst containing cloudy or hemorrhagic fluid. The wall of a large cyst may be several millimeters thick with an inner lining that is smooth or focally granular. The inner surface frequently is tan or brown, reflecting recent or old hemorrhage (Figure 11-146).

Intracystic carcinoma can have all of the architectural and cytologic appearances previously described for ductal carcinoma in situ (Figures 11-147 to 11-156). Most cases, however, have a papillary configuration (Figures 11-147, 11-148). Often there is a superimposed micropapillary and cribriform pattern (Figures 11-149, 11-150).

Regardless of the pattern of carcinoma, necrosis, with or without exfoliation of cells, may leave only a small component of identifiable neoplastic tissue. The recognizable tumor may be found along the cyst lining or floating free within the lumen. In either case, the usual cytologic and architectural criteria for ductal carcinoma in situ are applicable. Another trap that may lead to an underdiagnosis of intracystic carcinoma is the preservation of normal epithelium in some areas of the cyst wall. This is analogous to the presence of normal epithelium lining part of a duct containing either papillomas or ductal carcinoma in situ. The occurrence of large cysts lined by normal epithelium is rare under any circumstances. Even in the presence of fibrocystic changes, the cysts are usually lined by apocrine cells rather than normal epithelium. From a practical standpoint, one should be very concerned that any hemorrhagic cyst of the breast, especially when thick-walled and occurring in an elderly woman, is an intracystic carcinoma. When confronted with a large cyst lined by normal epithelium in a postmenopausal woman, many additional sections should be taken in the search for foci of papillary carcinoma.

A frequent concern when dealing with intracystic carcinoma is the inclusion of neoplastic epithelium within the duct or cyst wall, evidence that suggests invasion. Whether or not there is continuity of the intramural and intraductal components, a judgment regarding invasion can be difficult. We believe that as long as the epithelium does not conspicuously extend into the fat or stroma beyond the confines of the fibrous duct or cyst wall, it should be interpreted as entrapment of noninvasive carcinoma.

Intraductal Mucinous Carcinoma

Ductal carcinoma in situ is rarely associated with abundant mucin formation (Figure 11-157). The epithelium lining the duct may be effaced and the mucin may abut the underlying stroma. Most carcinomas with mucin production consist of a population of small cells that may contain minimal intracytoplasmic mucin (Figure 11-158). The differential diagnosis of mucinous carcinoma includes mucocele-like lesions in which there is no recognizable epithelial abnormality (Figure 11-159). There may be a histiocytic response to the mucin (Figure 11-160). Occasionally, normal-appearing cells line the mucocele-like duct (Figures 11-161, 11-162). In the absence of neoplastic cells, a diagnosis of carcinoma cannot be made based on the presence of mucin alone. Multiple sections should be taken, however, as mucocele-like lesions are sometimes associated with either mucinous carcinoma or atypical hyperplasia (Ro et al).

REFERENCES

Andersen JA, Nielsen M, Blichert-Toft M. The growth pattern of in situ carcinoma in the female breast. *Acta Oncologica* 1988;27:739-743.

Azzopardi JG. *Problems in Breast Pathology*. WB Saunders Co, Philadelphia, 1979, pp 192-239.

Betsill WL Jr, Rosen PP, Lieberman PH, Robbins GF. Intraductal carcinoma. Long-term follow-up after treatment by biopsy alone. *JAMA* 1978;239:1863-1867.

Broders AC. Carcinoma in situ contrasted with benign penetrating epithelium. *JAMA* 1932;99:1670-1674.

Carter D, Orr SL, Merino MJ. Intracystic papillary carcinoma of the breast. After mastectomy, radiotherapy or excisional biopsy alone. *Cancer* 1983;52:14-19.

Carter D, Smith RRL. Carcinoma in situ of the breast. *Cancer* 1977;40:1189-1193.

Charpin C, Lissitzky JC, Jacquemier J, et al. Immunohistochemical detection of laminin in 98 human breast carcinomas. A light and electron microscopic study. *Hum Pathol* 1986;17:355-365.

Chaudary MA, Girling A, Girling S, et al. New lumps in the breast following conservation treatment for early breast cancer. *Breast Cancer Res Treat* 1988;11:51-58.

Clement PB, Young RH, Azzopardi JG. Collagenous spherulosis of the breast. *Am J Surg Pathol* 1987;11:411-417.

Elston CW, Ellis IO. Pathology and breast screening. *Histopathology* 1990;16:109-118.

Eusebi V, Foschini MP, Cook MG, et al. Long-term follow-up of in situ carcinoma of the breast with special emphasis on clinging carcinoma. *Semin Diagn Pathol* 1989;6:165-173.

Fentiman IS, Fagg N, Millis RR, Hayward JL. *In situ* ductal carcinoma of the breast. Implications of breast pattern and treatment. *Eur J Surg Oncol* 1986;12:261-266.

Fisher ER, Brown R. Intraductal signet ring carcinoma. A hitherto undescribed form of intraductal carcinoma of the breast. *Cancer* 1985;55:2533-2537.

Fisher ER, Sass R, Fisher B, et al. Pathologic findings from the National Surgical Adjuvant Breast Project (Protocol 6). I. Intraductal carcinoma (DCIS). *Cancer* 1986;57:197-208.

Grignon DJ, Ro JY, Mackay BN, et al. Collagenous spherulosis of the breast. Immunohistochemical and ultrastructural studies. *Am J Clin Pathol* 1989;91:386-392.

Guerry P, Erlandson RA, Rosen PP. Cystic hypersecretory hyperplasia and cystic hypersecretory duct carcinoma of the breast. Pathology, therapy and follow-up of 39 patients. *Cancer* 1988;61:1611-1620.

Gump FE, Jicha DL, Ozello L. Ductal carcinoma in situ (DCIS). A revised concept. *Surgery* 1987;102:790-795.

Haupt HM, Rosen PP, Kinne DW. Breast carcinoma presenting with axillary lymph node metastases. An analysis of specific histopathologic features. *Am J Surg Pathol* 1985;9:165-175.

Jensen RA, Page DL. Cystic hypersecretory carcinoma. What's in a name? *Arch Pathol Lab Med* 1988;112:1179 (letter).

Kerner H, Lichtig C. Lobular cancerization. Incidence and differential diagnosis with lobular carcinoma in situ of breast. *Histopathology* 1986;10:621-629.

Koenig C, Vazquez M, Vohra R, Roses D. Subclassification of intraductal carcinoma as a guide to therapy. *Mod Pathol* 1990;3:53A.

Lagios MD, Margolin FR, Westdahl PR, Rose MR. Mammographically detected duct carcinoma in situ. Frequency of local recurrence following tylectomy and prognostic effect of nuclear grade on local recurrence. *Cancer* 1989;63:618-624.

Lagios MD, Westdahl PR, Margolin FR, Rose MR. Duct carcinoma *in situ*. Relationship of extent of noninvasive disease to the frequency of occult invasion, multicentricity, lymph node metastases, and short-term treatment failures. *Cancer* 1982;50:1309-1314.

Lagios MD. Human breast precancer. Current status. *Cancer Surveys* 1983;2:383-402.

Lagios MD, Westdahl PR, Rose MR. The concept and implications of multicentricity in breast carcinoma. *Pathol Annu* 1981;16(part 2):83-102.

Meyer JS. Cell kinetics of histologic variants of *in situ* breast carcinoma. *Breast Can Res Treat* 1986;7:171-180.

Millis RR, Thynne GSJ. *In situ* intraduct carcinoma of the breast. A long term follow-up study. *Br J Surg* 1975;62:957-962.

Page DL, Anderson TJ. *Diagnostic Histopathology of the Breast.* Churchill Livingstone, Edinburgh, 1987, p 279.

Page DL, Dupont WD, Rogers LW, Landenberger MA. Intraductal carcinoma of the breast. Follow-up after biopsy only. *Cancer* 1982; 49: 751-758.

Patchefsky AS, Schwartz GF, Finkelstein SD, et al. Heterogeneity of intraductal carcinoma of the breast. *Cancer* 1989;63:731-741.

Patchefsky AS, Shaber GS, Schwartz GF, et al. The pathology of breast cancer detected by mass population screening. *Cancer* 1977;40:1659-1670.

Ro J, Sahin A, Sneige N, et al. Mucocele-like tumor (MLT) of the breast. A clinicopathologic study of 6 cases. *Mod Pathol* 1990;3:83A.

Rosen PP, Senie R, Schottenfeld D, Ashikari R. Noninvasive breast carcinoma. Frequency of unsuspected invasion and implications for treatment. *Ann Surg* 1979;189:377-382.

Rosen PP. Axillary lymph node metastases in patients with occult noninvasive breast carcinoma. *Cancer* 1980;46:1298-1306.

Rosen PP, Braun DW Jr, Kinne DE. The clinical significance of pre-invasive breast carcinoma. *Cancer* 1980;46:919-925.

Rosen PP, Scott M. Cystic hypersecretory duct carcinoma of the breast. *Am J Surg Pathol* 1984;8:31-41.

Rosen PP. Mucocele-like tumors of the breast. *Am J Surg Pathol* 1986;10:464-469.

Sarnelli R, Squartini F. Multicentricity in breast cancer. A submacroscopic study. *Pathol Annu* 1986;21(part 1):143-158.

Schnitt SJ, Silen N, Sadowsky NL, et al. Ductal carcinoma in situ (intraductal carcinoma) of the breast. *N Engl J Med* 1988;318:898-903.

Schuh ME, Nemoto T, Penetrante RB, et al. Intraductal carcinoma. Analysis of presentation, pathologic findings, and outcome of disease. *Arch Surg* 1986;121:1303-1307.

Schwartz GF, Feig SA, Patchefsky AS. Significance and staging of nonpalpable carcinomas of the breast. *Surg Gynecol Obstet* 1988;166:6-10.

Schwartz GF, Patchefsky AS, Feig SA, et al. Multicentricity of non-palpable breast cancer. *Cancer* 1980;45:2913-2916.

Silverberg SG, Chitale AR. Assessment of significance of proportions of intraductal and infiltrating tumor growth in ductal carcinoma of the breast. *Cancer* 1973;32:830-837.

118   Tavassoli FA, Norris HJ. A comparison of the results of long-term follow-up for atypical intraductal hyperplasia and intraductal hyperplasia of the breast. *Cancer* 1990; 65: 518-529.

Walker AN, Fechner RE. Papillary carcinoma arising from ectopic breast tissue in an axillary lymph node. *Diagn Gynecol Obstet* 1982; 4: 141-145.

Webber BL, Heise H, Neifeld JP, Costa J. Risk of subsequent contralateral breast carcinoma in a population of patients with *in situ* breast carcinoma. *Cancer* 1981;47:2928-2932.

Wellings SR, Jensen HM, Marcum RG. An atlas of subgross pathology of the breast with special reference to possible precancerous lesions. *JNCI* 1975;55:231-273.

Zafrani B, Fourquet A, Vilcog JR, et al. Conservative management of intraductal breast carcinoma with tumourectomy and radiation therapy. *Cancer* 1986;57:1299-1301.

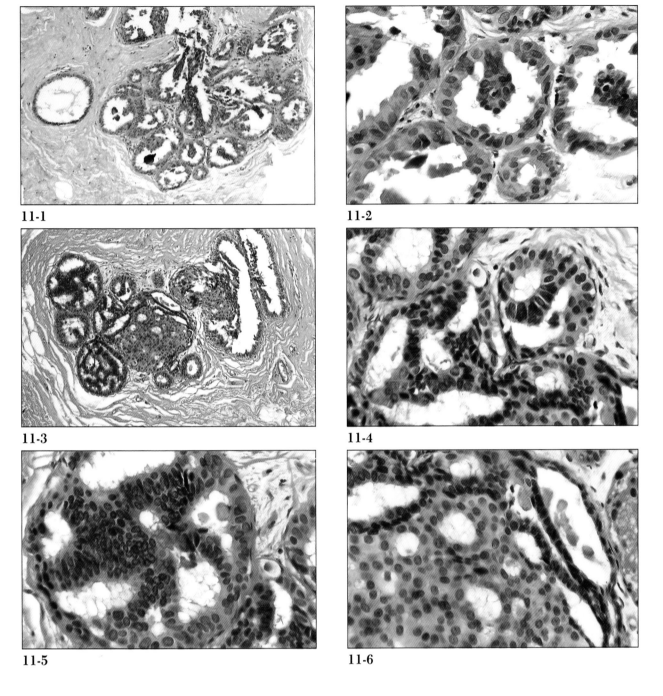

11-1

11-2

11-3

11-4

11-5

11-6

Figure 11-1. This partially unfolded lobule, from a patient with clear-cut ductal carcinoma in situ elsewhere, contains a markedly atypical epithelial proliferation with architectural features suggestive of micropapillary ductal carcinoma in situ. Whether this area is interpreted as ductal carcinoma in situ or severely atypical hyperplasia is arbitrary.

Figure 11-3. This unfolding lobule has architectural derangements mimicking both micropapillary and cribriform ductal carcinoma in situ. The interpretation of this field is arguable, although this specimen also contained unequivocal ductal carcinoma in situ elsewhere.

Figure 11-5. Another higher magnification of Figure 11-3 shows a central aggregate of benign-appearing cells with overlapping nuclei. Nonetheless, these bridges lack nuclear "streaming" and have a more rigid appearance.

Figure 11-2. A higher magnification of Figure 11-1 shows a small ductule (bottom) with irregularly distributed, small, benign-appearing nuclei typical of hyperplasia. The other ductules contain a mixed population of small, benign-appearing nuclei, as well as larger, pleomorphic, atypical forms.

Figure 11-4. A higher magnification of Figure 11-3 shows "rigid bridges." However, the epithelium includes both variably shaped, overlapping nuclei and areas of more evenly spaced cells with monomorphic nuclei.

Figure 11-6. Another higher magnification of Figure 11-3 demonstrates a predominantly monomorphic population of cells with lumen formation. Benign epithelial cells are also retained, especially at the left and in the right lower corner.

DUCTAL CARCINOMA IN SITU

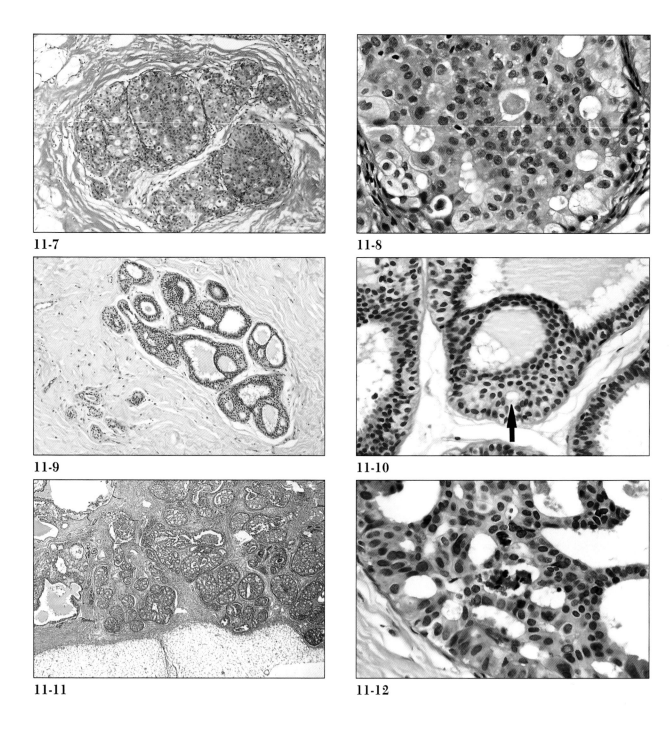

11-7

11-8

11-9

11-10

11-11

11-12

Figure 11-7. The enlarged ductules of this lobule are filled with atypical epithelium in a pattern resembling cribriform ductal carcinoma in situ. Unequivocal cribriform ductal carcinoma in situ was present elsewhere in the specimen.

Figure 11-9. This unfolding lobule contains ductules with a monomorphic cell population and architectural arrangements of both cribriform and micropapillary ductal carcinoma in situ.

Figure 11-11. This example of ductal carcinoma in situ has a large number of ducts per unit area. This can only be accounted for by the unfolding of adjacent lobules with progressive ductular enlargement.

Figure 11-8. A higher magnification of Figure 11-7 demonstrates that the spaces are partially surrounded by well-oriented cells, suggesting true lumina. The cytologically atypical cells have sharply defined cell borders.

Figure 11-10. A higher magnification of Figure 11-9 confirms the presence of a monomorphic cell population, despite the fact that there are occasional overlapping nuclei. The arrow indicates a true lumen.

Figure 11-12. A higher magnification of Figure 11-11 shows a monomorphic population of cells with focal comedonecrosis.

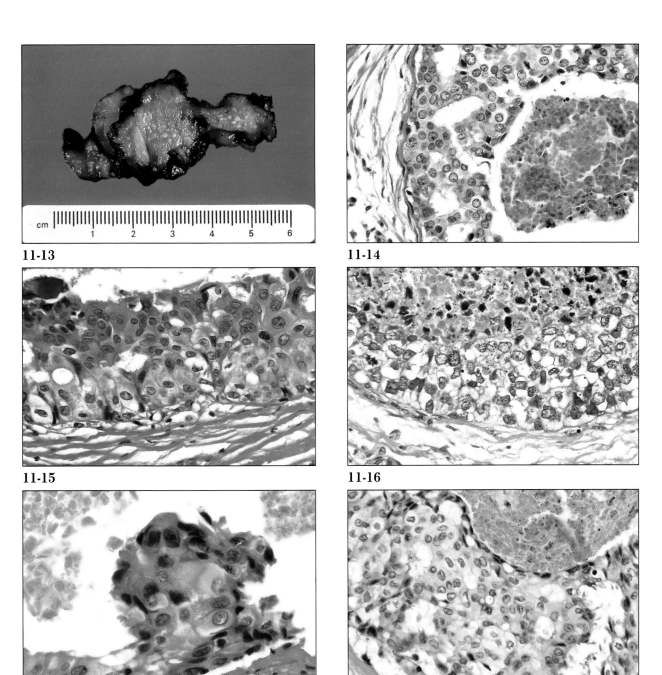

11-13

11-14

11-15

11-16

11-17

11-18

Figure 11-13. The cut surface of this breast specimen shows multiple light yellow nodules representing the necrosis-filled ducts of comedocarcinoma.

Figure 11-15. In this example of comedocarcinoma, the neoplastic cells form a more solid layer lining the involved duct. A few smaller, elongated nuclei are interspersed among the neoplastic cells and may represent residual normal epithelium.

Figure 11-17. Large, pleomorphic cells with abundant eosinophilic cytoplasm suggest apocrine differentiation in this comedocarcinoma.

Figure 11-14. The cells at the periphery of comedocarcinoma may have an irregular distribution, resulting in spaces that appear to be true lumina. The cells are moderately large and exhibit considerable cytologic uniformity.

Figure 11-16. Another example of comedocarcinoma is populated by cells having a high nuclear-to-cytoplasmic ratio and predominantly clear cytoplasm.

Figure 11-18. Often, the innermost layer of epithelium in comedocarcinoma is flattened and slightly separated from the necrotic debris.

DUCTAL CARCINOMA IN SITU

122

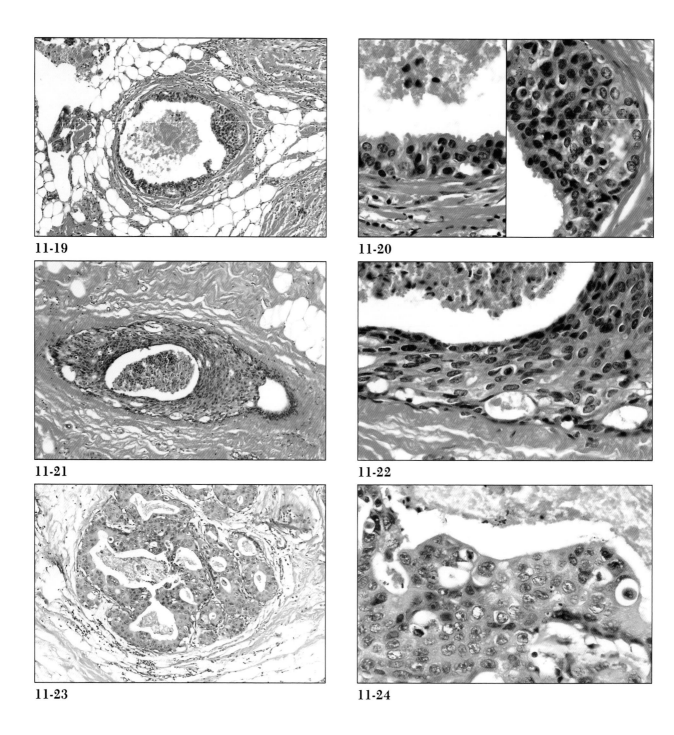

11-19

11-20

11-21

11-22

11-23

11-24

Figure 11-19. The cells of comedocarcinoma are occasionally minimally atypical.

Figure 11-21. This example of comedo-carcinoma has cells with minimal atypia and compression of the cells nearest the lumen. A remnant of the normal duct epithelium is seen at the right.

Figure 11-23. Seemingly complex epithelial proliferations in comedocarcinoma may be due to the involvement of multiple, closely apposed ductules, as well as larger ducts.

Figure 11-20. Higher magnifications of Figure 11-19 show minimally atypical epithelium.

Figure 11-22. A higher magnification of Figure 11-21 shows a flattened luminal layer of epithelial cells. The underlying neoplastic cells have only minimal cytologic atypia.

Figure 11-24. A higher magnification of Figure 11-23 shows cells with vesicular nuclei and individual cell necrosis.

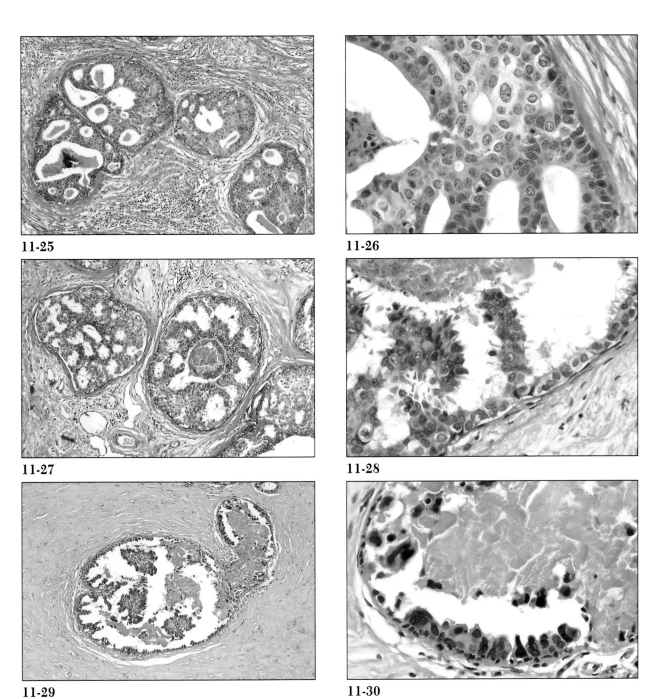

11-25

11-26

11-27

11-28

11-29

11-30

Figure 11-25. Some intraductal carcinomas have a combination of micropapillary and cribriform architecture with necrosis, as seen here. Whether these are viewed as comedo-carcinoma or micropapillary/cribriform ductal carcinoma in situ with necrosis is arbitrary.

Figure 11-27. Ductal carcinoma in situ with a more complex papillary architecture may also have small foci of necrosis. As in the previous case, the diagnostic terminology applied to this carcinoma is arbitrary.

Figure 11-29. Ducts involved with comedo-carcinoma may have only a thin mural layer of neoplastic cells.

Figure 11-26. A higher magnification of Figure 11-25 shows only slight cellular pleomorphism. The cells are of approximately the size seen in micropapillary/cribriform carcinoma.

Figure 11-28. A higher magnification from the same case as Figure 11-27 shows small cells with minimal atypia forming a right-angle papilla characteristic of micropapillary ductal carcinoma in situ.

Figure 11-30. A higher magnification of Figure 11-29 shows a thin layer of markedly pleomorphic cells. There is full-thickness necrosis of the epithelium at the right. A myoepithelial cell layer is present for most of the ductal circumference.

DUCTAL CARCINOMA IN SITU

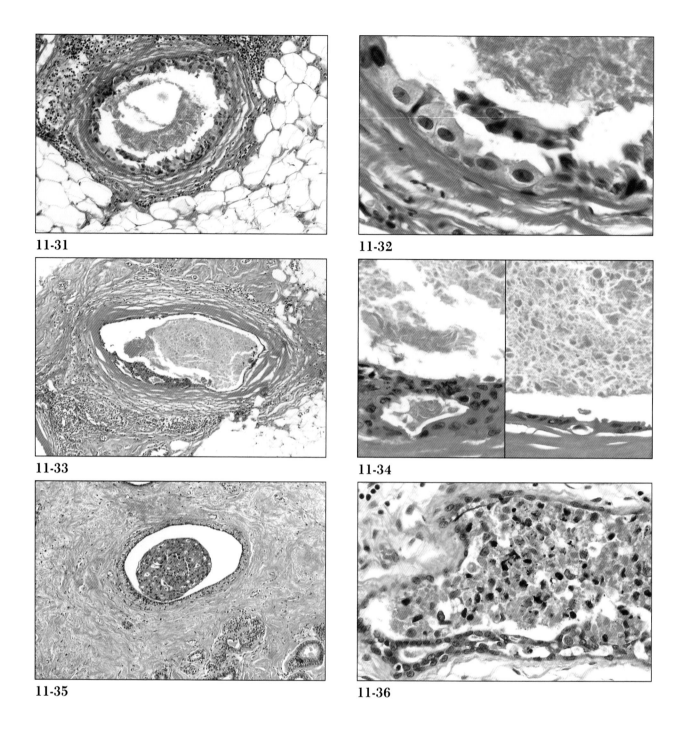

11-31

11-32

11-33

11-34

11-35

11-36

Figure 11-31. The thin layer of neoplastic epithelium in some examples of comedo-carcinoma may be composed of more uniform cells resembling lobular carcinoma in situ.

Figure 11-33. This example of comedocarcinoma has minimal periductal elastosis. Most of the epithelium is a single layer.

Figure 11-35. Comedocarcinoma may manifest as "embolized" atypical cells and necrotic debris in an otherwise typical duct.

Figure 11-32. A higher magnification of Figure 11-31 shows cells with a few well-defined cell borders and powdery cytoplasm.

Figure 11-34. Higher magnifications of Figure 11-33 show that part of the epithelium has small, lumen-like spaces containing necrotic debris (left). The single layer of presumably neoplastic epithelium is attenuated (right).

Figure 11-36. Comedocarcinoma may be intermixed with cytologically bland, mildly hyperplastic cells. The only evidence of carcinoma is the extensive necrosis and atypical exfoliated epithelium.

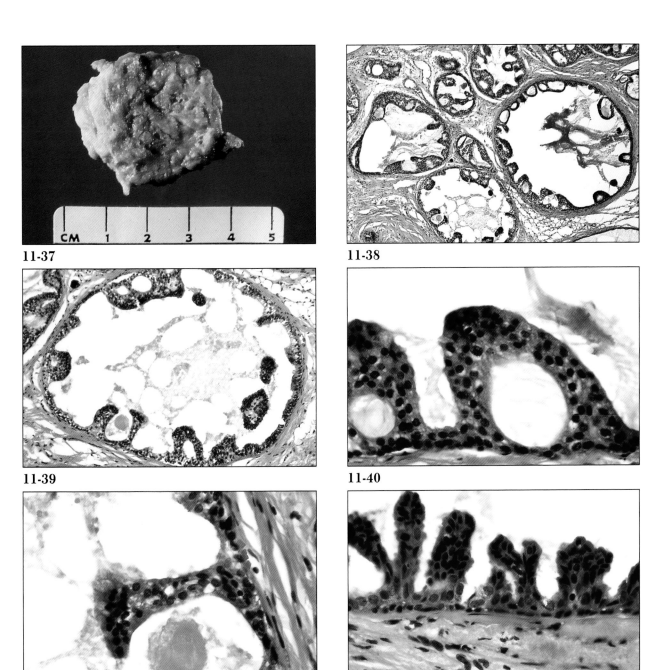

11-37

11-38

11-39

11-40

11-41

11-42

Figure 11-37. The cut surface of this biopsy specimen containing micropapillary ductal carcinoma in situ has ducts with grossly visible lumina. In other areas, a granular appearance is due to ducts filled with epithelial cells and debris.

Figure 11-39. A higher magnification of Figure 11-38 shows a duct with epithelial bridges and papillae of neoplastic cells. The eosinophilic material in the lumen is secretory and not necrotic debris, as is seen in comedocarcinoma.

Figure 11-41. The papillae of micropapillary ductal carcinoma in situ are also composed of a monomorphic population of cells. The tip of the papilla is often widened, in contrast to the papillae of hyperplasia.

Figure 11-38. A microscopic section from the lesion seen in Figure 11-37 shows closely approximated ducts and smaller ductules containing ductal carcinoma in situ.

Figure 11-40. The bridges of micropapillary ductal carcinoma in situ are composed of a monomorphic population of cells. There is no "streaming" of the epithelial cells within the bridge.

Figure 11-42. The papillae of micropapillary ductal carcinoma in situ may assume various shapes and sizes, including branching structures. Although some of the nuclei are elongated and appear to be "streaming," this is a monomorphic population of cells. A myoepithelial cell layer is clearly visible.

DUCTAL CARCINOMA IN SITU

126

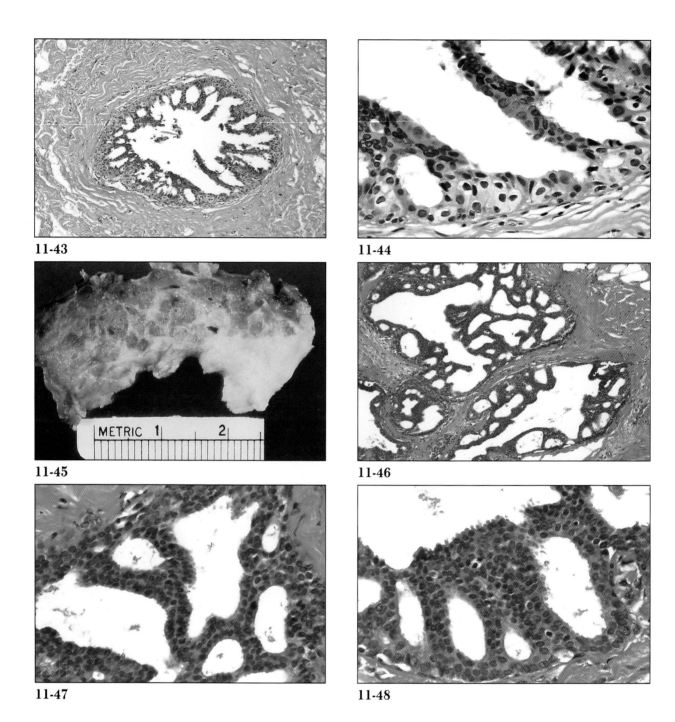

11-43

11-44

11-45

11-46

11-47

11-48

Figure 11-43. This example of micropapillary ductal carcinoma in situ has larger, well-preserved neoplastic cells at the periphery and progressively smaller neoplastic cells centrally. This results in a "pseudopagetoid" appearance.

Figure 11-45. This resection specimen containing micropapillary ductal carcinoma in situ has widely dilated, tan ducts filled with neoplastic epithelium.

Figure 11-47. A higher magnification of Figure 11-46 shows complex epithelial proliferations. For the most part, the nuclei are evenly spaced and the cells are oriented along the lumina without "streaming."

Figure 11-44. A higher magnification of Figure 11-43 shows degenerative changes in the intraluminal neoplastic component, manifested predominantly as smaller cells with denser eosinophilic cytoplasm. This is most conspicuous at upper right.

Figure 11-46. The closely apposed ducts of micropapillary ductal carcinoma in situ have lumina almost filled with neoplastic cells, accounting for the gross appearance in Figure 11-45.

Figure 11-48. Micropapillary ductal carcinoma in situ often consists of neoplastic epithelium forming adjacent broad bridges with resultant lumina. The apocrine "snouts" seen here are of no diagnostic value.

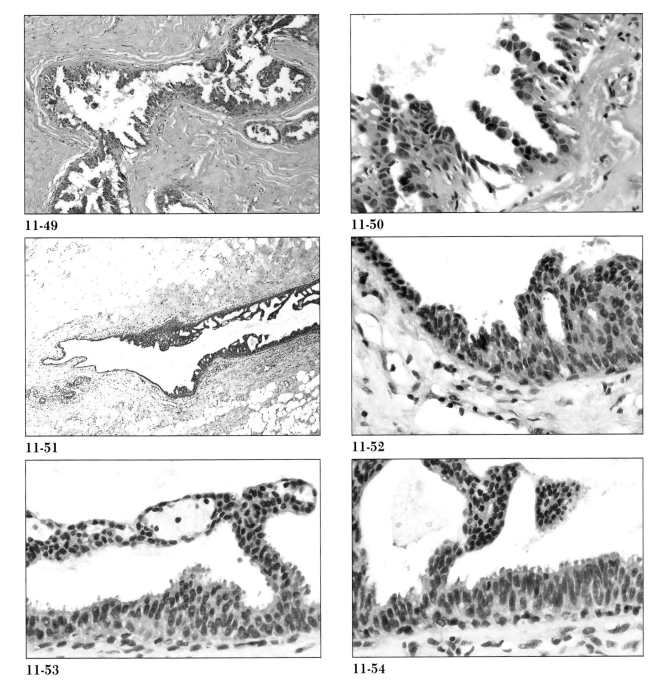

11-49

11-50

11-51

11-52

11-53

11-54

Figure 11-49. In this example of micropapillary ductal carcinoma in situ the papillae vary from broad structures to delicate forms composed of a narrow layer of cells.

Figure 11-51. This large, subsegmental duct is partially involved with micropapillary ductal carcinoma in situ. A broad range of papillary patterns is apparent. Figures 11-52 to 11-54 are higher magnifications of this duct.

Figure 11-53. Despite some nuclear variability and overlapping, the "rigid" appearance of the intraluminal epithelium supports the diagnosis of micropapillary ductal carcinoma in situ. The foamy histiocytes intermixed with the epithelium are of no diagnostic importance.

Figure 11-50. A higher magnification from Figure 11-49 shows that the narrow papillae are composed of neoplastic cells that have a "pavement stone" configuration.

Figure 11-52. The normal double layer of the duct at the left abuts the neoplastic component at the right. In this junctional region there is nuclear overlapping and a diagnosis of carcinoma would be difficult to make on this field, taken out of context.

Figure 11-54. The elongated, pseudostratified cells at the periphery contrast with the smaller, cuboidal cells of the distal portion of the papilla. This tendency for intraluminal cells to be smaller than their counterparts closer to the basement membrane is typical of many epithelial proliferations. This is not the polymorphism of hyperplasia.

DUCTAL CARCINOMA IN SITU

128

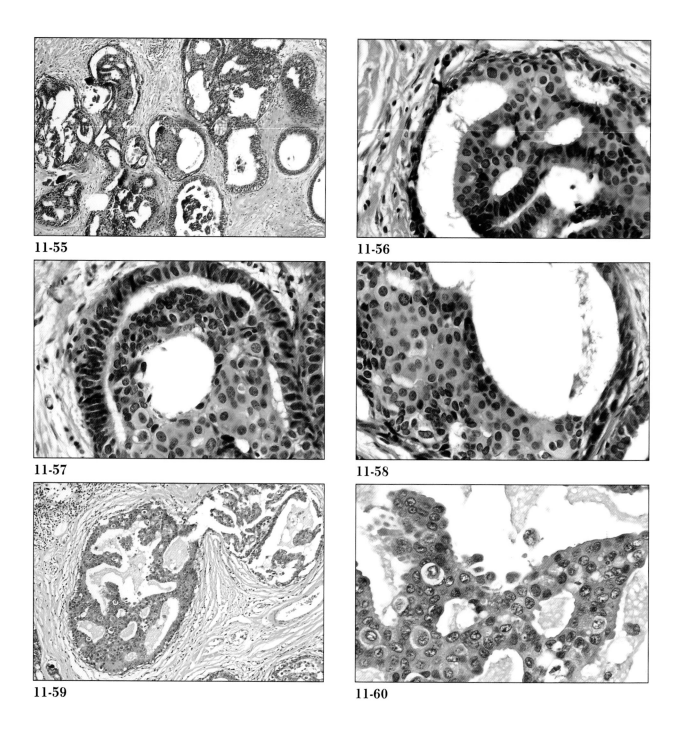

11-55

11-56

11-57

11-58

11-59

11-60

Figure 11-55. The complex epithelial patterns in this low-power magnification represent multiple ducts that are partially involved by micropapillary ductal carcinoma in situ, as seen at higher magnification in Figures 11-56 to 11-58.

Figure 11-57. This annular arrangement of intraductal epithelium has a monomorphic component of neoplastic cells in its lower half. The upper portion is composed of an apparently polymorphic population resembling hyperplasia.

Figure 11-59. This micropapillary ductal carcinoma in situ has vertical papillations and complex bridges. The presence of considerable secretory material in the lumina should heighten the suspicion of carcinoma.

Figure 11-56. The apparently normal ductal epithelium at the left merges with ductal carcinoma in situ at the top of the duct. The epithelial bridges appear to be composed of two populations of neoplastic cells.

Figure 11-58. A broad sheet of epithelial cells includes monomorphic neoplastic forms. The cells lining the duct (right) and the cells seen at lower left are not recognizable as neoplastic.

Figure 11-60. This higher magnification of Figure 11-59 shows neoplastic epithelial cells with atypical, moderately pleomorphic, vesicular nuclei. The occasional apocrine-like cytoplasmic "snouts" may be related to the secretory luminal material. Although there are ovoid, overlapping nuclei, this is a qualitatively monomorphic cell population.

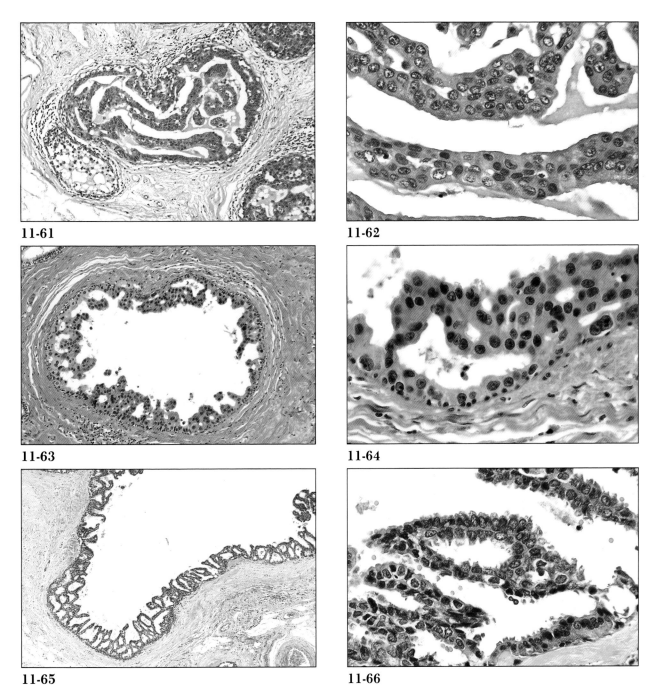

11-61

11-62

11-63

11-64

11-65

11-66

Figure 11-61. This example of micropapillary ductal carcinoma in situ has long papillary bridges of epithelium. The cells forming the papillae are identical to those lining the duct wall.

Figure 11-63. The typical papillary configuration of micropapillary ductal carcinoma in situ is populated by cells with dense nuclei and deeply eosinophilic cytoplasm.

Figure 11-65. This example of micropapillary ductal carcinoma in situ demonstrates both complex papillary bridges and isolated, right-angle papillae.

Figure 11-62. A higher magnification of Figure 11-61 demonstrates that a few elongated, small, bland nuclei are present within the lower papilla. Nonetheless, the architecture is that of carcinoma and most of the cells form a monomorphic population.

Figure 11-64. A higher magnification of Figure 11-63 shows epithelial cells with apocrine-type, eosinophilic cytoplasm. Paradoxically, most of the neoplastic cells have smaller, denser nuclei than those usually seen in apocrine metaplasia.

Figure 11-66. A higher magnification of Figure 11-65 shows moderately large, vesicular nuclei with a high nuclear-to-cytoplasmic ratio.

130

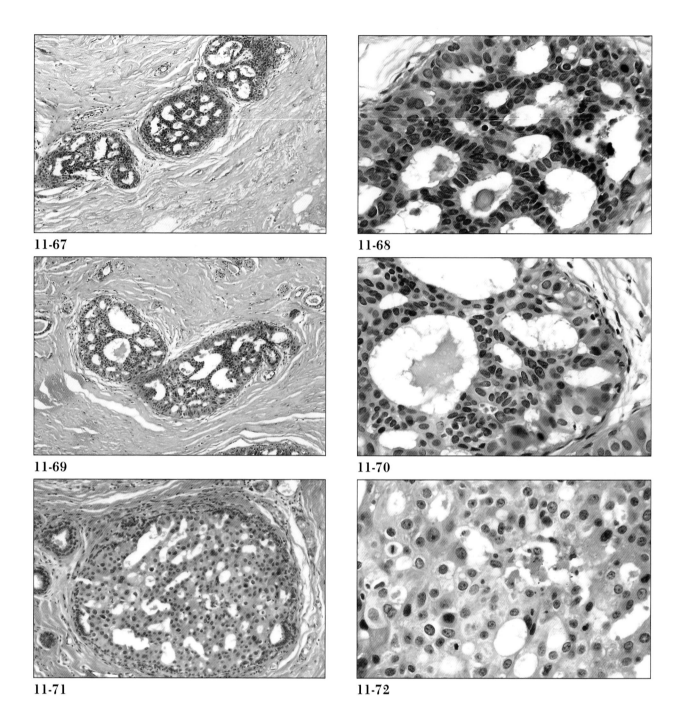

11-67

11-68

11-69

11-70

11-71

11-72

Figure 11-67. These ducts contain micropapillary ductal carcinoma in situ with extensive, transluminal bridges.

Figure 11-69. This example of micropapillary ductal carcinoma in situ exhibits cytologic variation seen at higher magnification in Figure 11-70.

Figure 11-71. This micropapillary ductal carcinoma in situ almost completely fills the duct and leaves irregular lumen-like spaces, mimicking the architecture of florid hyperplasia. Residual, normal ductal epithelium is present peripherally at the left and right sides of the duct.

Figure 11-68. A higher magnification of Figure 11-67 shows larger neoplastic cells peripherally and smaller cells centrally. This results in a bimorphic appearance, although intermediate-sized cells are also present. These features suggest that a monomorphic population is present with the superimposed luminal cell change described in Figure 11-44.

Figure 11-70. A higher magnification of Figure 11-69 shows variably sized cells, perhaps reflecting multiple monomorphic cell populations. Moderately large, polygonal cells are at the periphery of the duct; the bridges are formed by smaller cells with scant cytoplasm.

Figure 11-72. A higher magnification of Figure 11-71 shows cells with qualitatively identical cytoplasmic staining and considerable nuclear variation. The small, central amount of detritus suggests ductal carcinoma in situ.

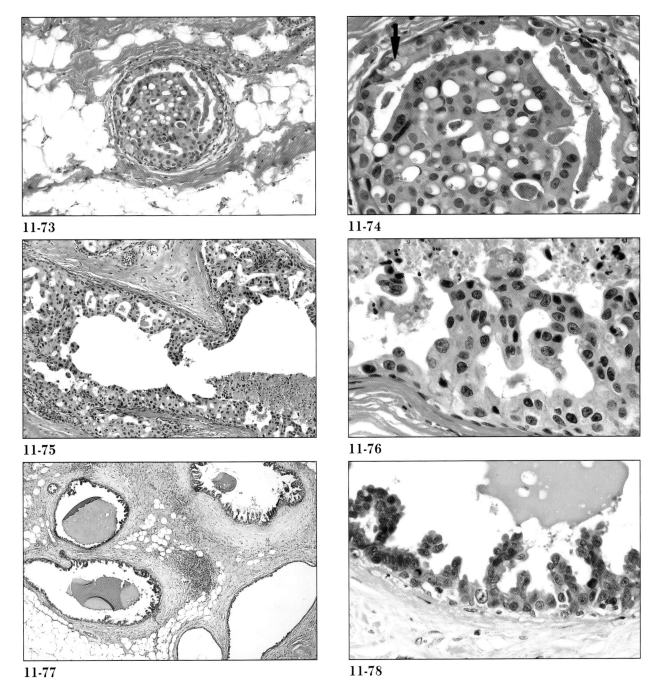

11-73

11-74

11-75

11-76

11-77

11-78

Figure 11-73. Another example of micropapillary carcinoma has eosinophilic cells with complex bridging.

Figure 11-75. A duct from the same case as illustrated in Figure 11-63 has the same general architecture but, in addition, there is a focus of comedo-type necrosis at the lower right.

Figure 11-77. So-called hypersecretory carcinoma is considered by some authors as a variant of micropapillary ductal carcinoma in situ that contains dense, eosinophilic, intraluminal secretions.

Figure 11-74. A higher magnification of Figure 11-73 discloses that several cells have clear spaces within the cytoplasm and compression of the adjacent nucleus. A few contain inspissated secretions, resulting in the appearance of a "target cell" (arrow).

Figure 11-76. A higher magnification of Figure 11-75 confirms the presence of degenerating cells in continuity with necrotic debris. The flattened nuclei of the well-preserved myoepithelial layer are conspicuous at the bottom of the illustration.

Figure 11-78. A higher magnification of Figure 11-77 shows that the moderately pleomorphic, neoplastic cells have minimal amounts of cytoplasm. Only the intraluminal secretion distinguishes this image from other patterns of micropapillary ductal carcinoma in situ.

DUCTAL CARCINOMA IN SITU

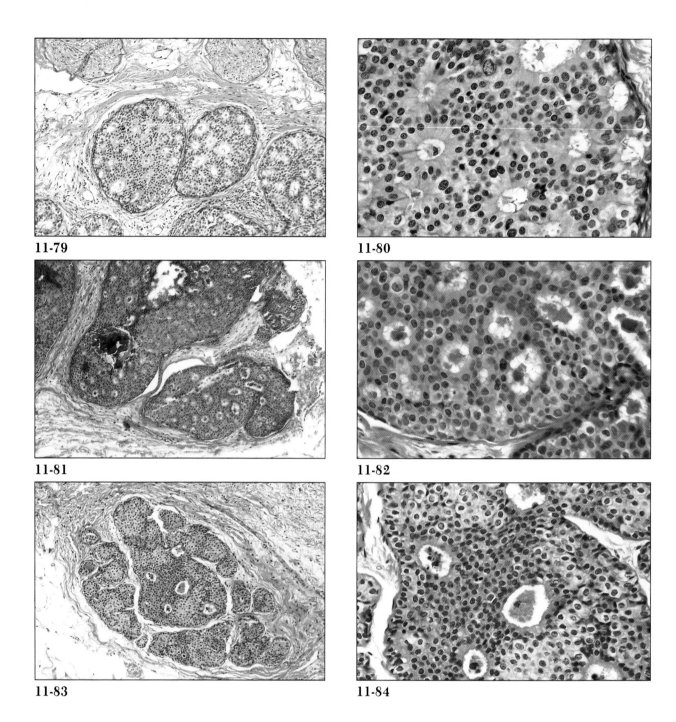

11-79

11-80

11-81

11-82

11-83

11-84

Figure 11-79. The ducts of cribriform ductal carcinoma in situ contain neoplastic cells that make well-formed, true lumina.

Figure 11-81. This example of cribriform ductal carcinoma in situ retains a central lumen (top). The associated microcalcification is of no diagnostic value.

Figure 11-83. The lobular origin of cribriform ductal carcinoma in situ is occasionally obvious when the involved ducts are small and have a lobular configuration, as seen here.

Figure 11-80. A higher magnification of Figure 11-79 shows an essentially monomorphic population of neoplastic epithelial cells. The presence of rare larger cells does not detract from this interpretation. The neoplastic cells are radially oriented around spaces, forming true glandular lumina.

Figure 11-82. A higher magnification of Figure 11-81 demonstrates cuboidal to low columnar cells lining the lumina, in contrast to the tall columnar cells seen in Figure 11-81. Intraluminal secretions are prominent and some are associated with microcalcifications (upper right).

Figure 11-84. A higher magnification of Figure 11-83 shows the well-oriented periluminal cells typical of cribriform ductal carcinoma in situ. Variation in the quantity of individual cell cytoplasm is evident in this monomorphic population.

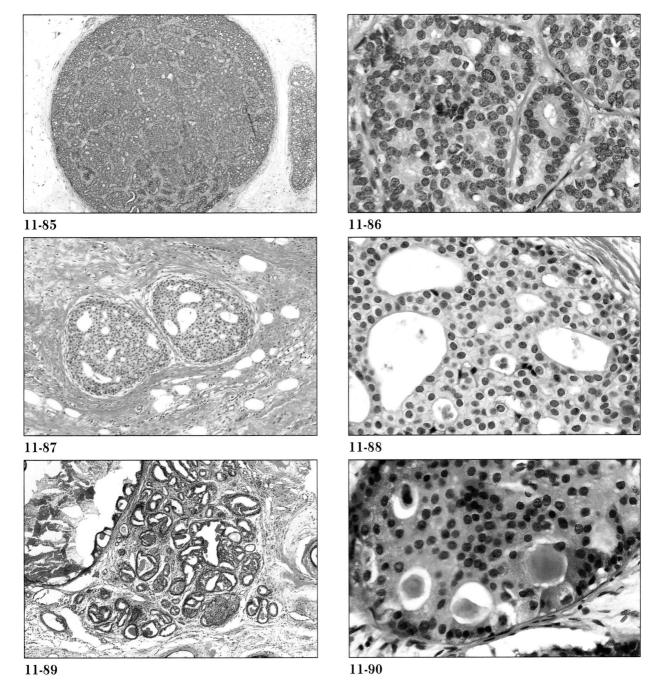

11-85

11-86

11-87

11-88

11-89

11-90

Figure 11-85. This markedly distended duct resembles a ductal adenoma at low magnification. Many lumina are discernible. Ducts of this size may have fibrovascular septa, as seen here, separating aggregates of cribriform carcinoma.

Figure 11-87. Cribriform ductal carcinoma in situ may occasionally consist of cells that are less well oriented around more irregularly shaped lumina.

Figure 11-89. Cribriform ductal carcinoma in situ is frequently associated with micropapillary ductal carcinoma in situ.

Figure 11-86. A higher magnification of Figure 11-85 shows neoplastic cells radially oriented around true lumina. Delicate fibrous septa separate the nests of cribriform carcinoma. As in Figure 11-80, the presence of occasional larger cells does not negate the interpretation that this is a monomorphic population.

Figure 11-88. A higher magnification of Figure 11-87 demonstrates that, although the neoplastic cells are haphazardly oriented around lumina, they are a monomorphic population. Cell borders are easily discerned.

Figure 11-90. A higher magnification of Figure 11-89 confirms the presence of round lumina typical of cribriform ductal carcinoma in situ.

DUCTAL CARCINOMA IN SITU

134

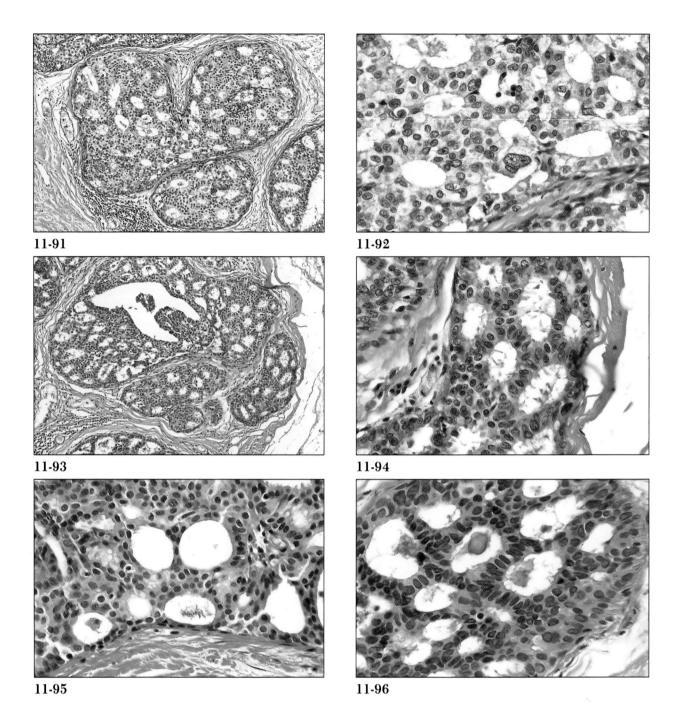

11-91

11-92

11-93

11-94

11-95

11-96

Figure 11-91. When ductal carcinoma in situ contains many lumina of varying shapes and sizes separated by only a few neoplastic cells, the distinction between cribriform and micropapillary variants becomes arbitrary.

Figure 11-93. Many of the lumina on the left are irregularly shaped and the architecture is suggestive of micropapillary ductal carcinoma in situ. On the right are rounder, more evenly spaced lumina, suggestive of cribriform ductal carcinoma in situ.

Figure 11-95. This intraductal proliferation has slightly irregular, lumen-like spaces. Some of the spaces are partially lined by well-oriented cells. Although this mimics cribriform ductal carcinoma in situ, the cell population is not monomorphic.

Figure 11-92. A higher magnification of Figure 11-91 demonstrates that the periluminal cells are less well oriented than in typical cribriform ductal carcinoma in situ.

Figure 11-94. A higher magnification of the right-hand portion of Figure 11-93 shows lumina separated by a layer of one or two cells. This can be interpreted as either cribriform or micropapillary ductal carcinoma in situ.

Figure 11-96. This intraductal proliferation lacks a monomorphic cell population and has lumen-like spaces only focally lined by apparently well-oriented cells. Based on these features, we interpret this as atypical ductal hyperplasia.

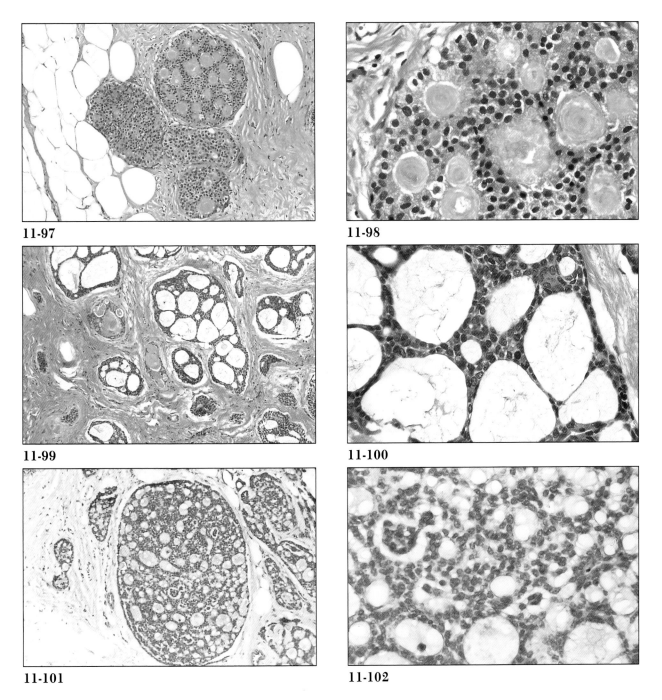

11-97

11-98

11-99

11-100

11-101

11-102

Figure 11-97. Intraductal collagenous spherulosis mimics cribriform ductal carcinoma in situ at low magnification. The eosinophilic material in the lumen-like spaces resembles the secretory material seen in cribriform carcinoma.

Figure 11-99. Adenoid cystic carcinoma may resemble both cribriform and micropapillary ductal carcinoma in situ at low magnification.

Figure 11-101. Another example of adenoid cystic carcinoma has numerous lumen-like spaces closely resembling cribriform ductal carcinoma in situ at low magnification. The irregularity of the smaller cellular nests suggests invasion and is characteristic of adenoid cystic carcinoma.

Figure 11-98. A higher magnification of Figure 11-97 shows amorphous eosinophilic extra-cellular material characteristic of collagenous spherulosis.

Figure 11-100. A higher magnification of Figure 11-99 demonstrates, however, that the cells of adenoid cystic carcinoma are basaloid and unoriented with respect to the pseudo-luminal spaces.

Figure 11-102. A higher magnification of Figure 11-101 confirms the basaloid nature of the neoplastic cells, as well as their nuclear overlapping and lack of orientation with respect to the pseudolumina.

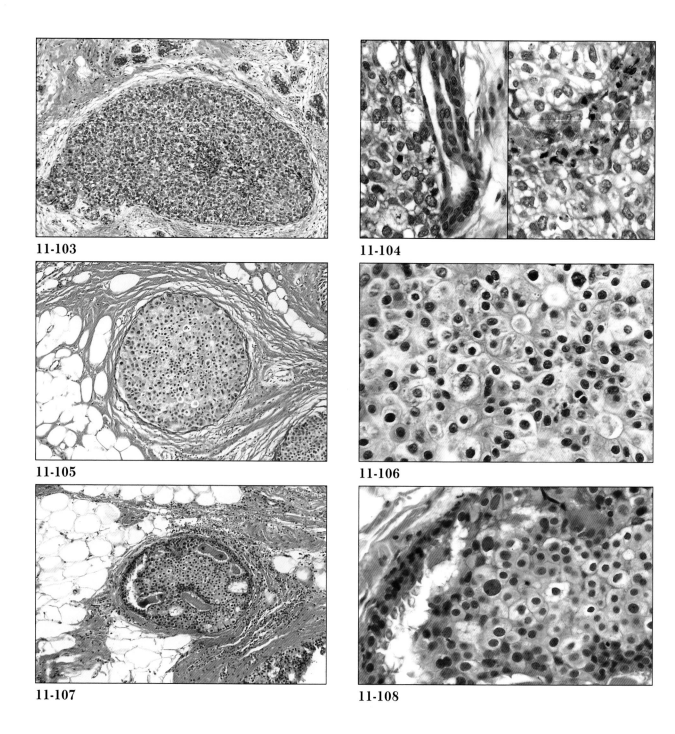

11-103

11-104

11-105

11-106

11-107

11-108

Figure 11-103. Solid ductal carcinoma in situ fills the duct with patternless sheets of neoplastic cells lacking necrosis or other more specific growth patterns. In this example, the cells are large with variably clear cytoplasm.

Figure 11-105. Solid ductal carcinoma in situ may have smaller cells with powdery eosinophilic cytoplasm. Compare this illustration with Figure 11-103.

Figure 11-107. In contrast to the previous examples, solid ductal carcinoma in situ need not completely fill the affected duct.

Figure 11-104. Some ducts containing solid ductal carcinoma in situ may have remnants of normal or hyperplastic epithelium at their peripheries (left). The example of solid ductal carcinoma in situ at the right contains necrotic cells in the central portion of the duct.

Figure 11-106. A higher magnification of Figure 11-105 shows a moderately pleomorphic cell population with a few lumina. This may be equally well interpreted as an unusually cellular variant of cribriform ductal carcinoma in situ.

Figure 11-108. A higher magnification of Figure 11-107 shows a monomorphic although moderately pleomorphic population of cells. Contrast the neoplastic cells with the normal epithelium lining the duct at the right.

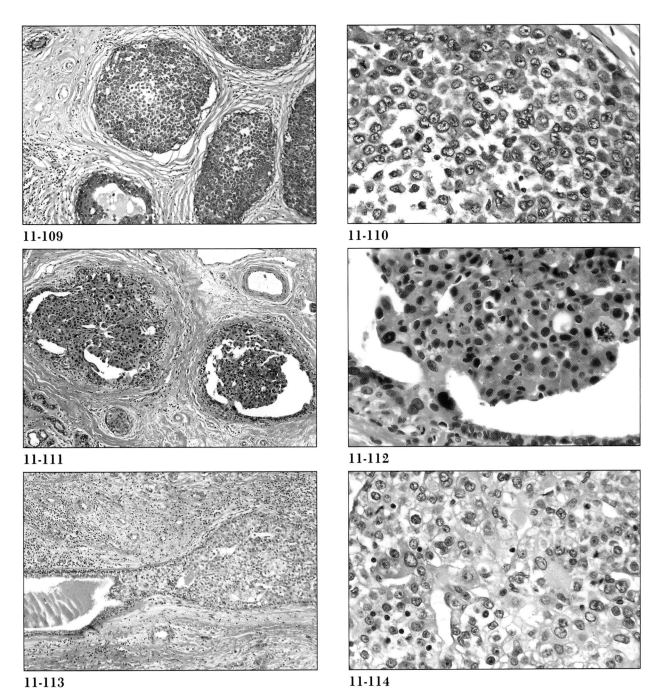

11-109

11-110

11-111

11-112

11-113

11-114

Figure 11-109. Another example of solid ductal carcinoma in situ has several ducts involved with loosely cohesive cells.

Figure 11-111. Some examples of solid ductal carcinoma in situ are not readily recognizable as malignant at low magnification. The peripherally located, irregular, lumen-like spaces seen here are more typical of hyperplasia.

Figure 11-113. This duct is partially involved with solid ductal carcinoma in situ. Although the architecture of the intraductal component suggests hyperplasia at this magnification, cytologically identical cells of infiltrating carcinoma are present at the top and bottom of the illustration.

Figure 11-110. A higher magnification of Figure 11-109 shows markedly abnormal nuclei and some degenerating cells (lower left).

Figure 11-112. A higher magnification of Figure 11-111 shows markedly abnormal cells and an atypical-appearing mitotic figure, justifying the diagnosis of solid ductal carcinoma in situ. Scattered necrotic cells are seen in the upper portion of the figure.

Figure 11-114. A higher magnification of Figure 11-113 shows severely atypical cells. There is a moderate amount of nuclear pleomorphism.

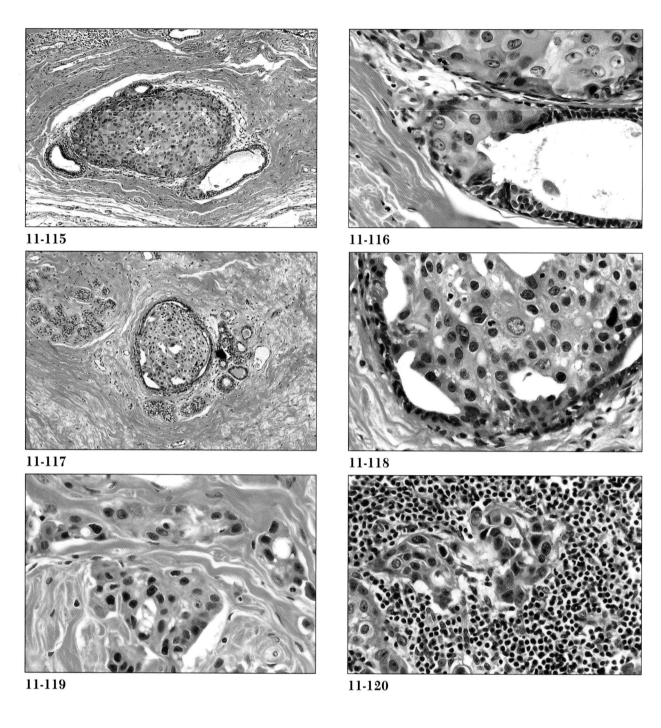

11-115

11-116

11-117

11-118

11-119

11-120

Figure 11-115. The central duct is completely filled with pleomorphic cells having large amounts of eosinophilic cytoplasm. The two adjacent ductules are partially involved with the same cells. We interpret this as solid ductal carcinoma in situ based on its cytologic identity with the infiltrating component from the same case shown in Figure 11-119.

Figure 11-117. Another duct from the case in Figures 11-115 and 11-116 is, presumably, an earlier stage in the development of solid ductal carcinoma in situ. The neoplastic epithelium is "tethered" to the duct wall in several foci.

Figure 11-119. Infiltrating carcinoma (same case as in Figures 11-115 through 11-118) has apocrine cells like the intraductal proliferations seen previously. Many cells have small, not recognizably malignant nuclei.

Figure 11-116. A higher magnification of Figure 11-115 shows apocrine-like neoplastic cells with vesicular nuclei and prominent nucleoli. Compare the sizes of the neoplastic nuclei and their normal counterparts lining the remainder of the ductule.

Figure 11-118. A higher magnification of Figure 11-117 shows that the normal ductal epithelium has been replaced by neoplastic cells at the points of attachment with the duct wall.

Figure 11-120. A lymph node metastasis from the same case shown in Figures 11-115 through 11-119 includes small as well as large cells. Several of the cells have coarse cytoplasmic vacuoles identical to those seen in Figures 11-117 and 11-119.

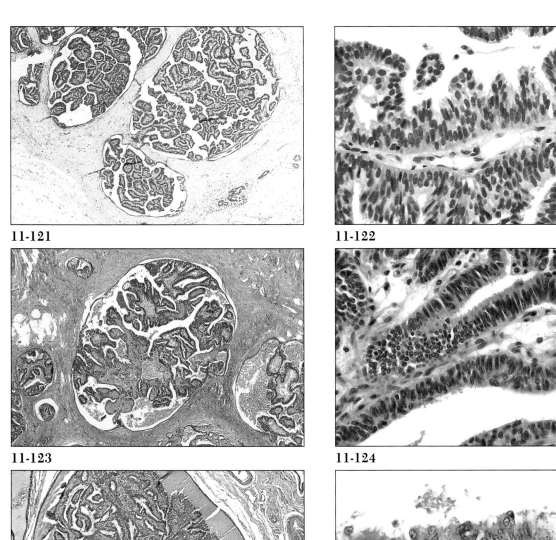

11-121

11-122

11-123

11-124

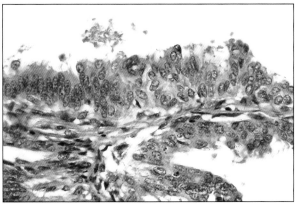

11-125

11-126

Figure 11-121. Papillary ductal carcinoma in situ is distinguished from other forms of ductal carcinoma in situ by the presence of fibrovascular stalks. In this example from deep within the breast, multiple ducts are involved.

Figure 11-123. This example of papillary ductal carcinoma in situ has hyalinized fibrovascular stalks, as are commonly seen in intraductal papillomas.

Figure 11-125. This example of papillary ductal carcinoma in situ in a large segmental duct has complex, branching fibrovascular stalks of varying width.

Figure 11-122. A higher magnification of Figure 11-121 shows pseudostratified layers of monomorphic cells with elongated nuclei. The complex papillae may appear as bridges or apparently dissociated cell nests in certain planes of section.

Figure 11-124. A higher magnification of Figure 11-123 shows pseudostratified neoplastic cells lining papillae. The elongated nature of the nuclei produces variations in nuclear shape in different planes of section, but the uniformity of the chromatin indicates that this is a monomorphic population.

Figure 11-126. A higher magnification of Figure 11-125 shows minimally pleomorphic cells with vesicular nuclei. The disorganized appearance of the epithelium results in a pseudostratified pattern.

DUCTAL CARCINOMA IN SITU

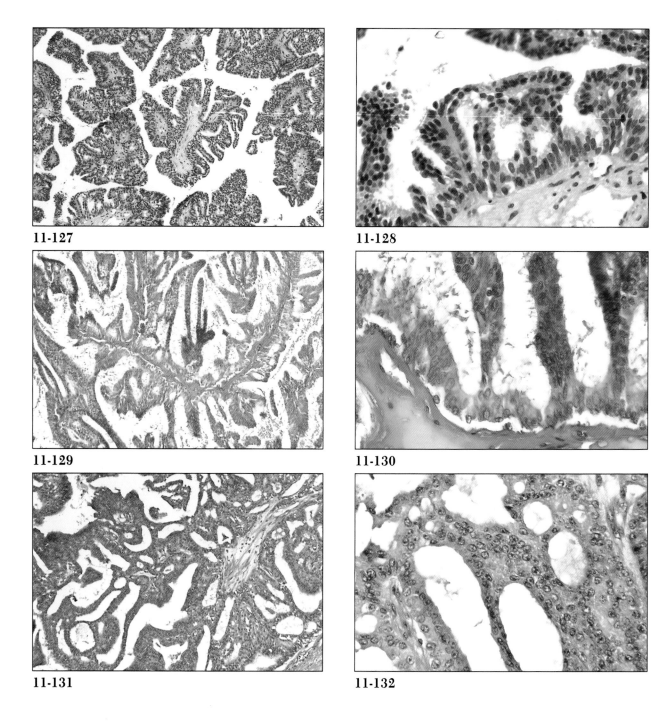

11-127

11-128

11-129

11-130

11-131

11-132

Figure 11-127. Papillary ductal carcinoma in situ may contain any of the other forms of ductal carcinoma in situ superimposed on the fibrovascular stalks. In this example, micropapillary forms are present.

Figure 11-129. This example of papillary ductal carcinoma in situ has many connecting papillae because of the complexity of the superimposed micropapillary component.

Figure 11-131. Another papillary carcinoma has florid superimposed micropapillary features, resulting in complex and irregularly shaped epithelial bridges.

Figure 11-128. This higher magnification of a fibrovascular stalk shown in Figure 11-127 is indistinguishable from typical micropapillary ductal carcinoma in situ.

Figure 11-130. A higher magnification of Figure 11-129 shows considerable variation in the size of chromatically uniform nuclei. We interpret this as a monomorphic cell population.

Figure 11-132. A higher magnification of Figure 11-131 discloses irregularly shaped lumen-like spaces lined by unoriented but cytologically uniform cells.

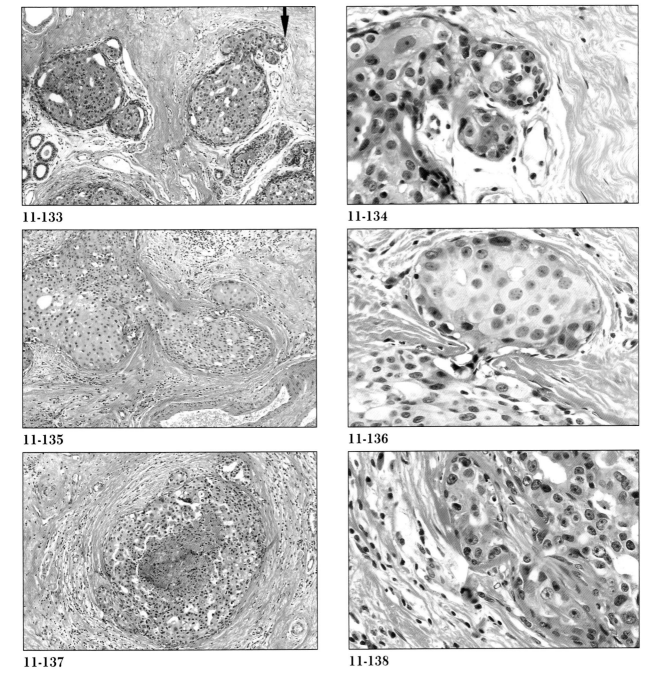

11-133

11-134

11-135

11-136

11-137

11-138

Figure 11-133. This example of solid ductal carcinoma in situ has irregular epithelial protrusions (arrow), suggesting microinvasion. Note, however, that there is no stromal reaction around the suspicious area.

Figure 11-135. This example of solid ductal carcinoma in situ has an epithelial protrusion that appears to be breaking through the fibrous stroma surrounding the large duct.

Figure 11-137. Comedocarcinoma has irregular nests of epithelial cells seemingly invading the stroma at lower right.

Figure 11-134. A higher magnification of Figure 11-133 shows a sharp epithelial-stromal junction with preservation of a few normal ductular epithelial cells. This is, thus, ductular extension, rather than microinvasion.

Figure 11-136. A higher magnification of Figure 11-135 shows a sharp epithelial-stromal junction. The collagen surrounding the protruding nest of cells is in continuity with and qualitatively similar to that surrounding the ducts.

Figure 11-138. A higher magnification of Figure 11-137 demonstrates nests of neoplastic cells sharply demarcated from the stroma by a narrow, circumferential band of collagen.

DUCTAL CARCINOMA IN SITU

142

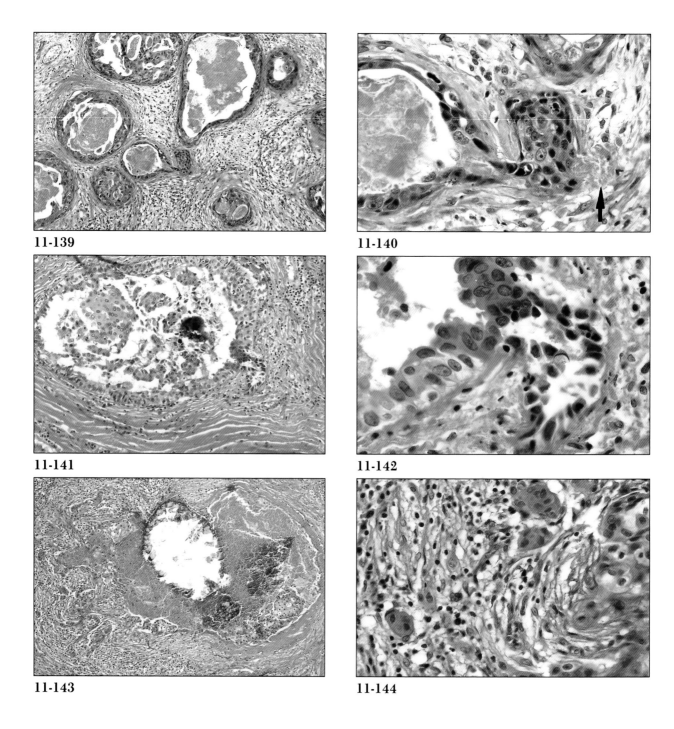

11-139

11-140

11-141

11-142

11-143

11-144

Figure 11-139. This example of comedocarcinoma has a loose fibrous stroma containing scattered lymphocytes. The irregularly shaped duct in the center suggests microinvasion.

Figure 11-141. Ductal carcinoma in situ has an angular protrusion of epithelium at the right. Again, the possibility of microinvasion is suggested.

Figure 11-143. The irregular contour of this duct with comedocarcinoma again raises the possibility of invasion. The fibrous stroma at the left is looser in appearance and contains more lymphocytes than the densely collagenous stroma at the right.

Figure 11-140. A higher magnification of Figure 11-139 shows blurring of the epithelial-stromal junction (arrow). Whether this is necrotic cytoplasmic debris from microinvasive carcinoma is uncertain. Such foci should not be interpreted as unequivocal microinvasion.

Figure 11-142. A higher magnification of Figure 11-141 shows that, despite the discohesive nature of the cells and their denser nuclei, the epithelial-stromal junction is sharp. This is not interpreted as microinvasion.

Figure 11-144. A higher magnification of the left side of Figure 11-143 shows small, dissociated nests of epithelial cells in a "fresh" fibroblastic reaction. The collagen is not circumferentially oriented around the cell nests. We interpret this as unequivocal microinvasion.

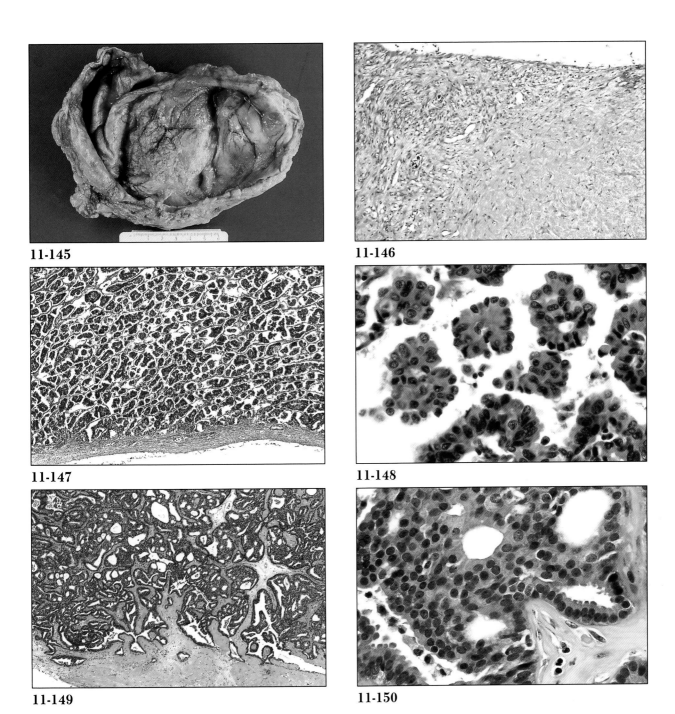

11-145

11-146

11-147

11-148

11-149

11-150

Figure 11-145. Intracystic carcinoma has a granular cyst lining in the central portion of the figure that contrasts with the predominantly smooth wall seen elsewhere.

Figure 11-147. The granularity of the cyst wall is caused by multiple foci of micropapillary carcinoma.

Figure 11-149. This example of intracystic carcinoma has a large component of fibro-vascular stalks. The epithelial component is a mixture of micropapillary and cribriform ductal carcinoma in situ.

Figure 11-146. Sections from the smooth portion of the cyst are devoid of epithelium. Recent hemorrhage in the cyst wall, as seen here, is common.

Figure 11-148. A higher magnification of Figure 11-147 shows apparently isolated papillae comprising a monomorphic population of cells that, nonetheless, exhibits some nuclear variation.

Figure 11-150. A higher magnification of Figure 11-149 includes a well-formed lumen typical of cribriform ductal carcinoma in situ.

DUCTAL CARCINOMA IN SITU

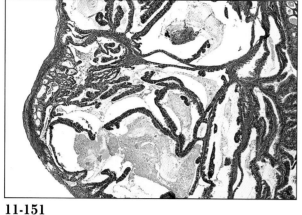

11-151

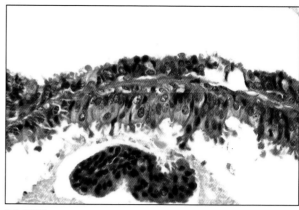

11-152

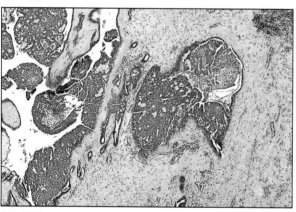

11-153

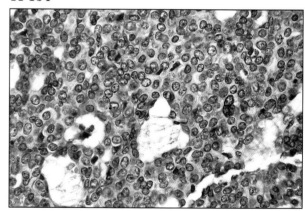

11-154

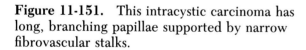

11-155

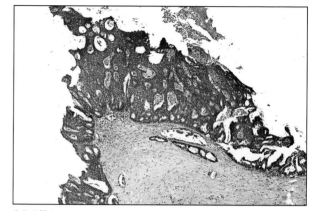

11-156

Figure 11-151. This intracystic carcinoma has long, branching papillae supported by narrow fibrovascular stalks.

Figure 11-153. Part of the cyst is lined by a flat layer of epithelium, and part has a micropapillary architecture. Hemorrhage and fibrosis are prominent within the wall.

Figure 11-155. Irregularities in the contour of intracystic carcinoma may, in some sections, result in seemingly isolated duct-like structures in the cyst wall. These should not be interpreted as invasive carcinoma or associated ductal carcinoma in situ outside of the cyst.

Figure 11-152. A higher magnification of Figure 11-151 shows a monomorphic population of atypical cells with enlarged, vesicular nuclei. These cells are intermixed with degenerating cells having small, dense nuclei. An aggregate of these degenerating cells appears to be free-floating in the lumen.

Figure 11-154. Another area of the tumor shown in Figure 11-153 has a thicker proliferation of papillary carcinoma. A normal duct is entrapped in the underlying fibrous tissue.

Figure 11-156. A higher magnification of the duct-like structure seen in Figure 11-155 illustrates ductal carcinoma in situ identical to that seen in the more obvious cyst lining.

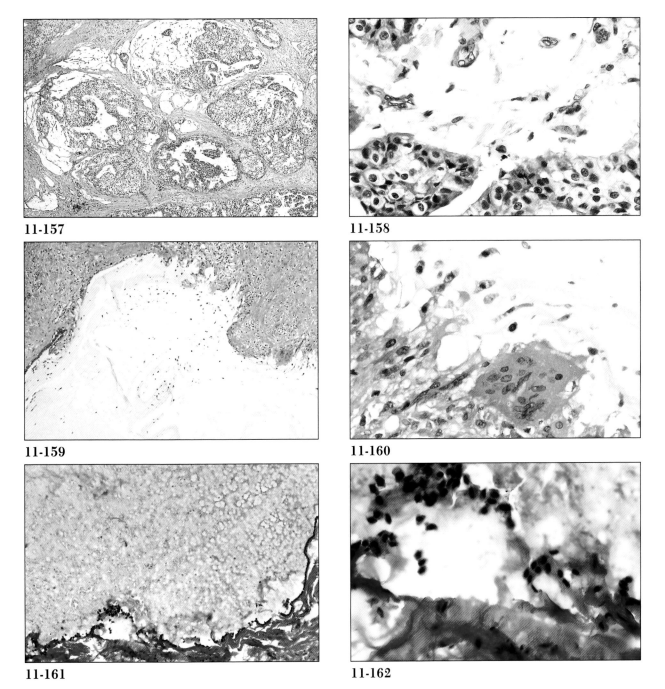

11-157

11-158

11-159

11-160

11-161

11-162

Figure 11-157. Micropapillary and cribriform ductal carcinoma in situ may produce large quantities of extracellular mucin. The mucin may penetrate the wall of the duct and infiltrate the surrounding stroma, as seen here, but this does not constitute invasive carcinoma.

Figure 11-159. Ductal carcinoma in situ must be distinguished from mucocele-like lesion of the breast, seen here. Some of the mucin-filled ducts may retain an intact, flattened epithelial lining (left). Other ducts have their epithelial lining replaced by histiocytes (right).

Figure 11-161. This example of mucocele-like change retains its epithelial lining.

Figure 11-158. A higher magnification of Figure 11-157 shows prominent extracellular mucin pooling with little evidence of intracytoplasmic mucin.

Figure 11-160. A higher magnification of Figure 11-159 shows that the lining epithelium of the cyst wall has been replaced by mononucleated and multinucleated histiocytes containing mucin. The free-floating cells are muciphages and not epithelial cells.

Figure 11-162. A higher magnification of Figure 11-161 shows that some of the benign epithelial cells have exfoliated into the mucin, and this should not be confused with mucinous carcinoma.

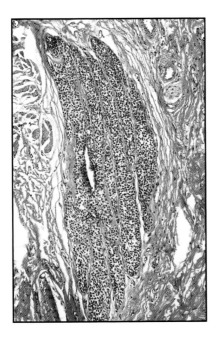

LOBULAR CARCINOMA IN SITU AND ATYPICAL LOBULAR HYPERPLASIA

12

Epithelial proliferations within the ductules of breast lobules span a wide spectrum of microscopic appearances. At one end of the spectrum are slightly enlarged ductules containing normal-appearing cells identical to those of ductal hyperplasia. At the other extreme are lobules containing ductules expanded by a monomorphic population of neoplastic cells typical of lobular carcinoma in situ. Lobular proliferations containing atypical cells lacking the full criteria for lobular carcinoma in situ are included under the term *atypical lobular hyperplasia*. As will be discussed, this term has slightly different definitions, depending on the authors who use it. Before applying risk data from a given study, one should be certain that the criteria applied to the case are appropriate. In some cases, our definition of atypical lobular hyperplasia differs slightly from that used by Page et al (1985) and, where appropriate, we have indicated that distinction.

LOBULAR CARCINOMA IN SITU

Foote and Stewart are generally credited with the first description of lobular carcinoma in situ in 1941, but illustrations dating back to the early 1900s show that others had recognized the lesion, using such terms as "acinar

carcinoma." Nonetheless, the publication by Foote and Stewart brought this entity into sharp focus. It was not until the late 1970s, however, that studies appeared documenting the clinical importance of lobular carcinoma in situ. When lobular carcinoma in situ appears as an incidental finding in a breast biopsy specimen, usually for fibrocystic changes, it places a woman at nine to 12 times greater risk for the development of invasive cancer as compared with the general population. In the premammographic era, approximately 33% of women with lobular carcinoma in situ in a biopsy specimen developed invasive cancer if the breast was left in place (Rosen et al). Fifty percent of the subsequent invasive cancers were in the contralateral breast.

The diagnosis of lobular carcinoma in situ is usually made in women from 35 to 55 years of age. However, it had been reported in the elderly in the premammographic era (Fechner, 1972), and it is unquestionably found frequently in mammogram-generated biopsy specimens from the elderly at the present time. Before mammography, approximately 1% to 3% of breast biopsy specimens obtained because of fibrocystic changes contained lobular carcinoma in situ as an incidental finding. In contrast, specimens from approximately 10% of mammogram-generated biopsies con-

148 tain lobular carcinoma in situ. Obviously, this statistic varies depending on the experience of the mammographer.

The term *lobular neoplasia* sometimes is used to identify a lesion morphologically identical to lobular carcinoma in situ. Cogent arguments can be mounted in support of both terms. Proponents of the term lobular carcinoma in situ correctly recognize the cytologic identity of infiltrating lobular carcinoma and its in situ counterpart. Antagonists note that an invasive carcinoma developing subsequent to lobular carcinoma in situ is more often an infiltrating large cell ductal carcinoma that does not resemble the previous lobular carcinoma in situ. Antagonists also point to the fact that a minority of patients with lobular carcinoma in situ who are left untreated (except by the initial biopsy) ever develop invasive carcinoma. This further supports the argument that lobular carcinoma in situ is not an obligatory malignancy during the life span of most women. Proponents of the term lobular neoplasia recognize this fact, and prefer the noncommittal, generic word "neoplasia," without judging whether the proliferating cells are benign or malignant. In our judgment, it is not crucial which term is used, as long as the clinical relevance is understood by the patient and her physician.

Before discussing the microscopic features of lobular carcinoma in situ, an important semantic problem must be addressed. The presence of large, ductal carcinoma-type cells in lobules raises the question of whether these cells represent lobular carcinoma in situ or so-called secondary cancerization of lobules by a ductal carcinoma. By convention, if there is an intraductal carcinoma composed of large cells, any lobular involvement by the same cells is viewed as cancerization and not as lobular carcinoma in situ. Obviously, there is continuity between the ductal system and the lobule, so it is not surprising that there should be overlap of microscopic features between different abnormal cells in both the lobular and ductal components of the breast. This concept is presented in greater detail on pages 151 and 152.

As we have discussed (page 110), the majority of mammary carcinomas arise from the terminal duct–lobular unit, whether they be small cell (lobular) or large cell (ductal) subtypes. As illustrated in Chapter 11, micropapillary and cribriform types of ductal carcinoma in situ are frequently encountered in slightly enlarged ductules derived from lobular unfolding. Lobular carcinoma in situ and

ductal carcinoma in situ sometimes coexist. Rosen et al found this combination in seven of 115 women with lobular carcinoma in situ. When these carcinomas involve large "ducts" and are thus defined as ductal carcinomas, they are often composed of cells cytologically identical to those of lobular carcinoma in situ. Thus, the current classification system for noninvasive ductal and lobular carcinomas produces semantic difficulties that sometimes complicate the discussion of what constitutes lobular carcinoma in situ and its distinction from ductal carcinoma in situ.

Despite the problems raised by the above issues, it is possible to place most lesions into diagnostic categories based on the size of the structure involved or the architecture of the epithelial proliferation. As we have illustrated, some cribriform and micropapillary architectural patterns are clearly located within ductules. We believe that these are best diagnosed as ductal carcinoma in situ, despite their location within a lobule. Conversely, the characteristic solid proliferation of lobular carcinoma in situ may greatly distend ductules to a size identical to small ducts. We prefer to diagnose these as lobular carcinoma in situ rather than a small cell solid ductal carcinoma in situ. Nonetheless, some structures are of intermediate size, making it impossible to decide whether they are very large ductules or very small ducts. In structures that are of indeterminate size, a problem exists when there is a predominately solid proliferation of small cells and rare lumina lined with well-oriented cells identical to cribriform carcinoma. Whether one considers this lobular carcinoma in situ with focal lumen formation or cribriform carcinoma with only rare lumen formation is arbitrary.

The problems just outlined are of limited clinical relevance. The risk for subsequent invasive carcinoma is similar, whether one calls a small cell tumor lobular carcinoma in situ or ductal carcinoma in situ. There is, however, one important caveat. Although the database is very small, it appears that ductal carcinoma in situ places the patient at a greater risk of developing cancer in the *ipsilateral* breast (Page et al, 1982). In contrast, lobular carcinoma in situ increases the risk of subsequent invasive carcinoma equally for both breasts. Rosen et al showed that the number of lobules with carcinoma in situ did not alter the risk for subsequent development of invasive cancer. In their study, the risk was the same whether a patient had only one involved lobule or more than 12 affected lobules in the first biopsy specimen.

In making the microscopic diagnosis of lobular carcinoma in situ, several different issues must be addressed. First, there are qualitative judgments regarding the cytologic changes. Lobular carcinoma in situ has a wide range of cytologic appearances that will be discussed momentarily. Having decided that the appropriate cytologic abnormalities are present, there are two questions regarding the quantity of cells necessary for the diagnosis. The problem of quantity begins with the number of atypical cells in an individual ductule that are required to render a diagnosis of lobular carcinoma in situ. Some authors require that the ductular lumen be completely obliterated and others require that the affected ductule be increased in diameter, whereas these are not criteria for still other observers.

The final quantitative diagnostic problem, assuming lobular distention as a criterion, is determining what proportion of ductules in a given lobule need be distended. Many authors believe that if the qualitative changes are sufficient for the diagnosis, all the ductules in a lobule need not be distended. However, Page et al (1985) require that more than one half of a lobule contain distended ductules before a diagnosis of lobular carcinoma in situ is warranted.

The presence of these individual cells resembling lobular carcinoma in situ raises a difficult diagnostic problem. In the broadest sense of the term, they represent atypical lobular hyperplasia. Nevertheless, there are no risk-assessment data available for the quantitatively few atypical cells seen in Figures 12-39 through 12-44.

Lobular carcinoma in situ is typically defined as a proliferation of monomorphic epithelial cells that are somewhat larger and slightly rounder than normal lobular cells. The neoplastic cells tend to be evenly spaced. The proliferation of cells usually obliterates the lumen of the involved ductule and distends its normal diameter. Mitotic figures are rarely found.

Against the backdrop of this idealized definition of lobular carcinoma in situ must be placed the reality of numerous cytologic variations. The cells of lobular carcinoma in situ, in fact, vary considerably in their nuclear and cytoplasmic features. This is partly acknowledged by some authors who designate the cell types of lobular carcinoma in situ as Type A and Type B. Type A cells have uniformly small, round, darkly staining nuclei with very small or absent nucleoli. Type B cells have larger nuclei with less uniform chromatin, and the nucleoli are often conspicuous. Between these two extremes are a heterogeneous group of intermediate-sized cells, often with a bubbly or vacuolated nucleus that presumably reflects an extremely irregular, convoluted shape.

The cytoplasm of the cells in lobular carcinoma in situ may be powdery and abundant. Such cells often have well-defined cell membranes. Other cells have only scant amounts of indistinct, poorly characterized cytoplasm. The latter cells have only a few, nondescript granules or strands of cytoplasm, and lack a recognizable cell membrane. In view of the nuclear and cytoplasmic variability of lobular carcinoma in situ, the diagnosis is uncommonly made solely by cytologic criteria. With the exception of the target cell to be described below, the only cytologically diagnostic cell has an enlarged, uniform nucleus, powdery cytoplasm, and well-demarcated cell margin. Ductules involved by these cells stand out sharply at low power because of the "pavement stone" appearance that this cell population imparts.

Part of the spectrum of lobular carcinoma in situ is illustrated in Figures 12-1 through 12-12. Cells can have small, evenly spaced nuclei and scant to modest amounts of cytoplasm (Figures 12-1 through 12-4). Although the neoplastic cells are usually closely packed (Figures 12-2, 12-4), they may also have a separated, discohesive appearance (Figure 12-5). Some cells with small nuclei have more abundant cytoplasm (Figure 12-6). Ductules can be populated by a mixture of small and large cells (Figures 12-7, 12-8). The larger cells tend to be more unevenly spaced, and they often lack recognizable cell borders (Figures 12-13, 12-14).

Other cytologic changes that may be encountered in lobular carcinoma in situ include effete or degenerating neoplastic cells having shrunken, uniformly hyperchromatic nuclei (Figures 12-11, 12-12). In other instances, the proliferating peripheral cells appear to compress and elongate the more centrally located nuclei (Figures 12-13, 12-14).

Lobules are sometimes located within fat and have virtually no intralobular fibrous stroma. When their component ductules are involved with lobular carcinoma in situ, they may mimic invasive carcinoma. The sharp circumscription and lack of stromal response in the surrounding adipose tissue distinguishes

150

such lobules from invasion (Figure 12-15). Rarely, squamous metaplasia is present as an incidental finding in lobular carcinoma (Figure 12-16).

One of the most distinctive cells in lobular carcinoma in situ is the target cell. The nucleus of a target cell may be round, but it is more often pushed to the side and slightly distorted by an intracytoplasmic lumen that appears as a sharply delimited, round, clear space (Figure 12-17). If there is secretion within this lumen, it forms an eosinophilic, dense, central droplet surrounded by an annular clear zone (Figure 12-18). The resultant image accounts for the name target cell. Ultrastructurally, the intracytoplasmic lumen is lined by a cell membrane that may have microvilli. The lumen is a totally enclosed sphere within the cell; the cell does not have the configuration of a doughnut. On rare occasions, a target cell will be seen in hyperplasia of the ordinary type or ductal carcinoma in situ. Therefore, it is not pathognomonic of lobular carcinoma in situ. Nevertheless, if more than a few target cells are seen within an epithelial proliferation, further sampling of the tissue, either by step sectioning of the block or submission of additional material, is warranted.

Approximately three fourths of cases of lobular carcinoma in situ have mucin in at least 25% of the tumor cells (Andersen and Vendelboe). Most of the mucin-positive cells are not recognizable as target cells, however. Mucin has been reported in 2% to 3% of ductal carcinomas that secondarily invaded the lobule (Gad and Azzopardi). Therefore, mucin-producing cells in the lobule favor a diagnosis of lobular carcinoma in situ, but they are not diagnostic.

Signet-ring cells are a rare form of lobular carcinoma in situ and are not the same as target cells. Signet-ring cells have an eccentric, compressed nucleus because the cytoplasm is almost completely filled with mucin. Ultrastructurally, there is no intracytoplasmic lumen.

Despite a broad cytologic spectrum, the diagnosis of lobular carcinoma in situ can be made if one judges that there is a *monomorphic* population of cells that has effaced the normal architecture of the ductule. Effacement of the normal architecture, in our opinion, requires total obliteration of the ductular lumen with distention of the ductular diameter.

Lobular carcinoma in situ can involve other architecturally distinctive lesions that are of lobular origin such as sclerosing adenosis (Figures 12-19 to 12-28). Usually, there is evidence of more clear-cut lobular carcinoma in situ elsewhere. The difficulty with lobular carcinoma involving sclerosing adenosis is its distinction from invasive carcinoma. The most helpful feature in this regard is the lack, in sclerosing adenosis, of the extreme stromal response with elastosis that is typical of infiltrating lobular carcinoma. Sclerosing adenosis usually has more dilated ductules or characteristic aggregates of cells at the periphery of the suspicious area. These peripheral ductules may be only partially involved with neoplasia (Figure 12-26). The overall architecture of sclerosing adenosis also can be identified if the section includes a central fibrous area that has a few uninvolved ductules (Figure 12-27).

Lobular carcinoma in situ involving large areas of sclerosing adenosis suggests the alveolar variant of infiltrating lobular carcinoma (Shousha et al). In contrast with sclerosing adenosis, however, the alveolar variant of infiltrating lobular carcinoma consists of well-defined aggregates of cells with a patternless arrangement scattered within fibrous stroma and fat (Figures 12-29, 12-30).

Differential Diagnosis

A number of alterations involving lobules can superficially mimic lobular carcinoma in situ. Clear cell change may obliterate most of a ductular lumen (Figure 12-31). The nuclei, however, are smaller, more elongated, and more variegated than those of lobular carcinoma (Figure 12-32). Architectural distortion or juxtaposition of lobules having clear cells can further complicate the interpretation (Figure 12-33), but attention to the cytologic features of clear cell change just described will allow distinction (Figure 12-34).

Epithelial hyperplasia of the usual type can completely fill and distend ductules (Figure 12-35). When the cells have ovoid nuclei and variable amounts of cytoplasm, they are easily distinguished from the monomorphic cell population of lobular carcinoma in situ (Figure 12-36). Rarely, cells in ductules have abundant eosinophilic and partly vacuolated cytoplasm similar to apocrine epithelium (Figures 12-37, 12-38). This apocrine-like change may involve a few ductules in lobules that elsewhere contain lobular carcinoma in situ (Eusebi et al).

Epithelial proliferations may distend ductules that still maintain their lumina (Figure 12-39). Alternately, the lumina may be ablated by a proliferation that includes cells with powdery cytoplasm characteristic of lobular carcinoma in situ, but with polymorphous nuclei identical to those of ordinary hyperplasia. There may also be cells with uniform, round nuclei that, coupled with the cytoplasm, become cytologically identical to the cells of lobular carcinoma in situ. When such cells are scattered among those having the appearance of ordinary hyperplasia, the criteria of lobular carcinoma in situ are not met (Figures 12-40 to 12-44). This leads to a problem regarding terminology. We refer to these cases as typical lobular hyperplasia. However, we recognize that this term is not to be used to assess risk, because such cases differ from those that Page et al (1985) termed atypical lobular hyperplasia in their risk-assessment studies. It should be recognized that many microscopically abnormal lobules do not fit any published pattern that has known risk for the subsequent development of invasive cancer.

Hyperplastic lobules may have a complex architecture because of closely apposed, irregular ductules, possibly intermixed with the intralobular portion of the terminal duct (Figure 12-43). This architectural irregularity does not mimic a form of ductal carcinoma in situ and, therefore, should not be considered to be atypical on architectural grounds. Such architecturally distorted foci may also contain scattered cells with the powdery cytoplasm or enlarged hyperchromatic nuclei of carcinoma in situ (Figure 12-44).

Another variant of atypical lobular hyperplasia consists of lobules containing a monomorphic population of cells qualitatively satisfactory for lobular carcinoma in situ, but lacking the quantitative criteria discussed above (Figures 12-45, 12-46). The involved ductules may have focal preservation of an inner lumen of normal epithelium (Figures 12-47 to 12-50). The proliferating cells may be small, intermediate, or large (Figures 12-51 to 12-60), just as in fully developed lobular carcinoma in situ. The monomorphic cells in this variant of atypical lobular hyperplasia may partially replace ductules, and maintain a sharp junction with the adjacent normal cells (Figures 12-61, 12-62). An especially vexing diagnostic problem is the lobule that has ductules totally populated by cells typical of lobular carcinoma in situ, including target cells, but lacking ductular enlargement (Fig-

ures 12-63, 12-64). We suspect that changes of the type illustrated in Figures 12-61 to 12-64 place the patient at the same risk for subsequent invasive carcinoma as the individual with fully diagnostic lobular carcinoma in situ, but, admittedly, we cannot prove this point.

Enlarged ductules populated by a mantle of monomorphic cells raise special problems of nomenclature (Figures 12-65, 12-66). The pattern of proliferation may be more suggestive of ductal carcinoma in situ than lobular carcinoma in situ. Nonetheless, the location within a lobule most logically places the lesion in the category of lobular neoplasia. The problem of lobular carcinoma in situ versus ductal carcinoma in situ becomes more complicated when there is maintenance of the lumen, and intraluminal debris raises the possibility of incipient comedonecrosis (Figures 12-67, 12-68). In the absence of clear-cut ductal carcinoma in situ (especially the comedocarcinoma pattern) elsewhere in the specimen, a diagnosis of atypical lobular hyperplasia must be made. When comedocarcinoma is identified in large ducts, the presence of necrotic debris in the lumina of ductules populated by atypical cells can be viewed as a component of ductal carcinoma in situ (Figures 12-69, 12-70). Occasionally, ductules involved with comedocarcinoma may be greatly distended and lined only by a few malignant cells (Figures 12-71, 12-72). Such areas may be easily overlooked at low magnification. Rare sections may demonstrate ductal carcinoma in situ contiguous with an involved lobule. In such instances, the interpretation of the lobular component is straightforward, especially when the ductal carcinoma is of the comedo type (Figures 12-73, 12-74). Usually, however, the affected lobule is not contiguous with an involved duct. One must then rely on pleomorphism, and the presence of lumina and intraluminal debris to recognize that the carcinoma in the lobule is ductal.

Even when there is comedocarcinoma and cytologically identical cells are present within a lobule, the question of simultaneous origin can be raised (Figures 12-75 to 12-78). If a ductule maintains its myoepithelial layer and has atypical cells replacing the inner layer, this strongly suggests that the abnormal cells are arising in situ as a field effect. Nonetheless, patient management is based on the diagnosis of the comedocarcinoma. Whether cytologically identical cells are arising in the ductules or extending into them is a moot point.

LOBULAR CARCINOMA IN SITU

Some carcinomas that involve the ducts and lobules are difficult to classify because they have features of both ductal and lobular carcinoma. Lobular carcinoma in situ may be clearly in continuity with ducts that have an identical population of small, uniform neoplastic cells (Figure 12-79). When the ductal component has architectural features of ductal carcinoma in situ, a combined diagnosis of lobular carcinoma in situ and ductal carcinoma in situ can be made, even though the population of cells is cytologically identical in both sites (Figures 12-79, 12-80). A greater diagnostic problem is presented when lobules and ducts in continuity are populated by cytologically identical cells that are larger and more pleomorphic than the usual cells of lobular carcinoma in situ (Figure 12-81). Since lobular carcinoma in situ can have large cells and a moderate degree of pleomorphism, the lobules taken out of context are indistinguishable from lobular carcinoma in situ (Figure 12-82). A pagetoid-like architecture in much of the ductal component further suggests lobular type neoplasia (see below) (Figure 12-83). However, when there is considerable cytoplasmic debris in the ductal lumen, such cases are probably better interpreted as lobular involvement by ductal carcinoma in situ resembling comedocarcinoma (Figure 12-84).

PAGETOID CHANGE

Cells identical to those of lobular carcinoma in situ can involve the epithelium of extralobular ducts, including the collecting ducts beneath the nipple. This phenomenon is often referred to as pagetoid spread of lobular carcinoma in situ, which implies that the cells originate in the ductules and grow into the duct system. Indeed, fortuitous sections may show abnormal cells in a lobule in continuity with cytologically identical pagetoid cells in a terminal duct (Figures 12-85, 12-86). In most instances, however, continuity cannot be demonstrated, either because it does not exist (see below), or because of the plane of sectioning.

Given the fact that some cases with so-called pagetoid spread lack lobular abnormalities, it seems preferable to refer to the presence of lobular carcinoma-type cells in extralobular ducts as pagetoid change, rather than spread. It is possible that in some or perhaps most instances, the abnormal cells are arising in these extralobular locations. This

may be true, even when there is fully typical lobular carcinoma in situ elsewhere in the breast. Furthermore, when lobular carcinoma in situ is contiguous with terminal ducts or larger ducts showing pagetoid change, it does not preclude a simultaneous proliferation of neoplastic cells in all of these sites.

Regardless of whether pagetoid change forms a single-cell or multicell layer in the ducts, the normal overlying epithelium is flattened (Figures 12-87, 12-88). The nuclei and cytoplasm of the preexistent normal epithelial cells are stretched out as a continuous layer over the tumor cells. The myoepithelial layer may be obvious, or difficult to identify. As long as there is no stromal invasion, it does not matter whether the outermost cells are pagetoid cells or myoepithelial cells. A sharp epithelial-stromal junction is sufficient evidence to exclude invasion.

The cells of pagetoid change may be intermixed with cells having elongated or round nuclei of smaller size. This results in a layer of epithelium that is several cells thick, probably representing a mixture of normal and neoplastic components. The neoplastic cells stand out because of their round shape, often enlarged nuclei, and sharp cell borders (Figures 12-89, 12-90).

Pagetoid change frequently forms a "cloverleaf pattern." The involved duct has sharply defined, often uniform, ovoid out-pouchings consisting of aggregates of neoplastic cells (Figures 12-91, 12-92). Only a sector of the duct may be involved. Usually, the entire circumference has evenly spaced out-pouchings. On rare occasions, the out-pouchings may be only a few cells wide, and are most easily identified when an adjacent normal duct is present for comparison.

Ducts with the cloverleaf pattern in cross-section can also be recognized when the duct is cut tangentially (Figures 12-93, 12-94). The parallel out-pouchings in a tangential section present a unique pattern that is easily identified at low magnification (Figure 12-95) and verified on cytologic grounds at higher power (Figure 12-96). Pagetoid change can involve the lactiferous ducts (Figures 12-97, 12-98) but, to our knowledge, Paget's disease of the nipple has never been described as a component of lobular carcinoma.

Pagetoid change can also involve ducts that contain other lesions. For example, we have seen pagetoid change of the walls of ducts that contained papillomas (Figures 12-99, 12-100). Rarely, the pagetoid cells extend partially onto the fronds of the papilloma with resultant flattening of the outermost benign epithelial cells.

The frequency with which pagetoid change is associated with lobular carcinoma in situ varies in different series. Andersen (1974) found lobular carcinoma in situ in all of the 41 cases of pagetoid change that he studied. However, in seven of his patients, additional sections were required to find the lobular lesion. On the other hand, Page et al (1988) found pagetoid change unassociated with lobular abnormalities in 66 women. In their retrospective study, they did not have the opportunity to submit additional material. Interestingly, these authors found that when pagetoid change occurred in the absence of atypical lobular hyperplasia it did not increase the risk for subsequent breast carcinoma. However, when it was associated with atypical lobular hyperplasia (Figures 12-87, 12-88), the risk for subsequent cancer rose to 6.8, a level intermediate between that of atypical lobular hyperplasia without pagetoid change (2.7 times) and that of lobular carcinoma in situ (ten to 11 times). Intuitively, pagetoid change should carry the same risk for invasive cancer as lobular carcinoma in situ, given Andersen's finding of lobular carcinoma in situ in all instances of pagetoid change. Although we are at a loss to explain the data reported by Page et al regarding this point, the large number of cases in their study provides strong support for their finding.

Foamy histiocytes within the epithelium may resemble pagetoid change at low magnification. At higher magnification the cytologic distinction is readily made. The nuclei of histiocytes are smaller than the cells of pagetoid change. There is more cytoplasm than in pagetoid cells, and it has a foamy appearance. The overlying normal epithelium is often flattened; a feature shared with pagetoid change (Figures 12-101, 12-102). Myoepithelial cells may have abundant clear cytoplasm and mimic the cells of pagetoid change. Myoepithelial cells, however, have small nuclei, often have a spindled shape, and usually form a single, even layer. They do not produce flattening of the overlying epithelium.

REFERENCES

Andersen JA. Invasive breast carcinoma with lobular involvement. Frequency and location of lobular carcinoma in situ. *Acta Pathol Microbiol Scand A* 1974;82:719-729.

Andersen JA. Lobular carcinoma in situ. A long-term follow-up in 52 cases. *Acta Pathol Microbiol Scand A* 1974;82:519-533.

Andersen JA. Lobular carcinoma in situ. A histological study of 52 cases. *Acta Pathol Microbiol Scand A* 1974;82:735-741.

Andersen JA. Lobular carcinoma in situ of the breast with ductal involvement. Frequency and possible influence on prognosis. *Acta Pathol Microbiol Scand A* 1974;82:655-662.

Andersen JA, Fechner RE, Lattes R, et al. Lobular carcinoma in situ. (Lobular neoplasia) of the breast (a symposium). *Pathol Annu* 1980; 15(part 1):192-223.

Andersen JA, Vendelboe ML. Cytoplasmic mucous globules in lobular carcinoma in situ. Diagnosis and prognosis. *Am J Surg Pathol* 1981; 5:251-255.

Breslow A, Brancaccio ME. Intracellular mucin production by lobular breast carcinoma cells. *Arch Pathol Lab Med* 1976;100:620-621.

Eusebi V, Betts C, Haagensen DE Jr, et al. Apocrine differentiation in lobular carcinoma of the breast. A morphologic, immunologic, and ultrastructural study. *Hum Pathol* 1984;15: 134-140.

Fechner RE. Ductal carcinoma involving the lobule of the breast. A source of confusion with lobular carcinoma in situ. *Cancer* 1971;28: 274-281.

Fechner RE. Epithelial alterations in the extralobular ducts of breasts with lobular carcinoma. *Arch Pathol* 1972;93:164-171.

Fechner RE. Lobular carcinoma *in situ* in sclerosing adenosis. A potential source of confusion with invasive carcinoma. *Am J Surg Pathol* 1981;5:233-239.

Foote FW Jr, Stewart FW. Lobular carcinoma in situ. A rare form of mammary cancer. *Am J Pathol* 1941;27:491-495.

Gad A, Azzopardi JG. Lobular carcinoma of the breast. A special variant of mucin-secreting carcinoma. *J Clin Pathol* 1975;28:711-716.

Haagensen CD, Lane N, Lattes R, Bodian C. Lobular neoplasia (so-called lobular carcinoma *in situ*) of the breast. *Cancer* 1978;42:737-769.

Haagensen CD, Lane N, Bodian C. Coexisting lobular neoplasia and carcinoma of the breast. *Cancer* 1983;51:1468-1482.

Page DL, Dupont WD, Rogers LW. Ductal involvement by cells of atypical lobular hyperplasia in the breast. A long-term follow-up study of cancer risk. *Hum Pathol* 1988;19: 201-207.

Page DL, Dupont WD, Rogers LW, Rados MS. Atypical hyperplastic lesions of the female breast. A long-term follow-up study. *Cancer* 1985;55:2698-2708.

154   Page DL, Dupont WD, Rogers LW, Landenberger M. Intraductal carcinoma of the breast. Follow-up after biopsy only. *Cancer* 1982; 49: 751-758.

Rosen PP, Lieberman PH, Braun DW Jr, et al. Lobular carcinoma in situ of the breast. Detailed analysis of 99 patients with average follow-up of 24 years. *Am J Surg Pathol* 1978; 2:225-251.

Shousha S, Backhouse CM, Alaghband-Zadeh J, Burn I. Alveolar variant of invasive lobular carcinoma of the breast. A tumor rich in estrogen receptors. *Am J Clin Pathol* 1986;85: 1-5.

Wheeler JE, Enterline HT. Lobular carcinoma of the breast in situ and infiltrating. *Pathol Annu* 1976;11:161-188.

Wheeler JE, Enterline HT, Roseman JM, et al. Lobular carcinoma in situ of the breast. Long-term followup. *Cancer* 1974;34:554-563.

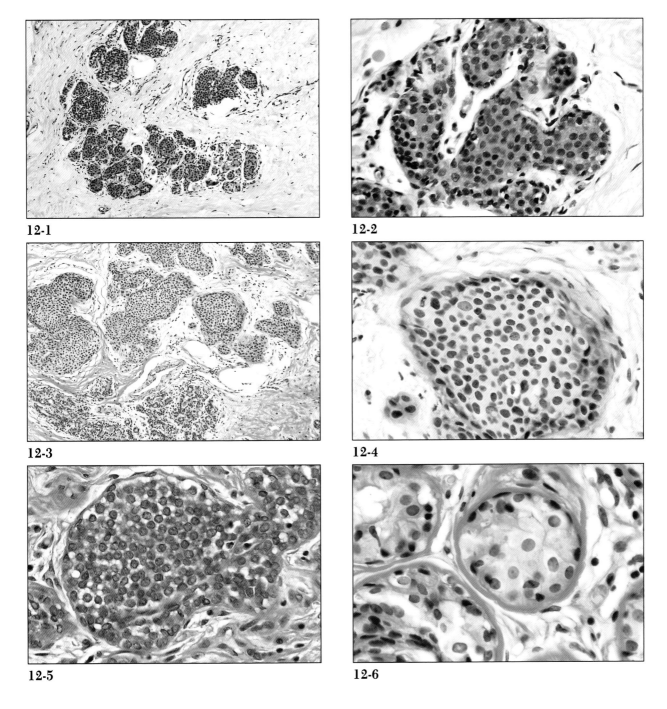

12-1

12-2

12-3

12-4

12-5

12-6

Figure 12-1. This example of lobular carcinoma in situ involves minimally dilated ductules.

Figure 12-3. This more florid example of lobular carcinoma in situ involves ductules that vary from minimally to widely dilated.

Figure 12-5. This example of lobular carcinoma in situ consists of cells with scant cytoplasm and unrecognizable cell borders.

Figure 12-2. A higher magnification of Figure 12-1 discloses that the ductules are filled with a single population of small cells exhibiting only slight cytologic variation.

Figure 12-4. A higher magnification of Figure 12-3 shows a slightly pleomorphic population of larger neoplastic cells, as compared with Figure 12-2. The mitotic figure at upper left is a very rare finding in lobular carcinoma in situ. The four neoplastic cells at lower left are not microinvasive carcinoma.

Figure 12-6. This lobular carcinoma in situ consists of cells with abundant, powdery cytoplasm and distinct cell borders. A few myoepithelial cells with spindled nuclei are compressed at the periphery of the ductule.

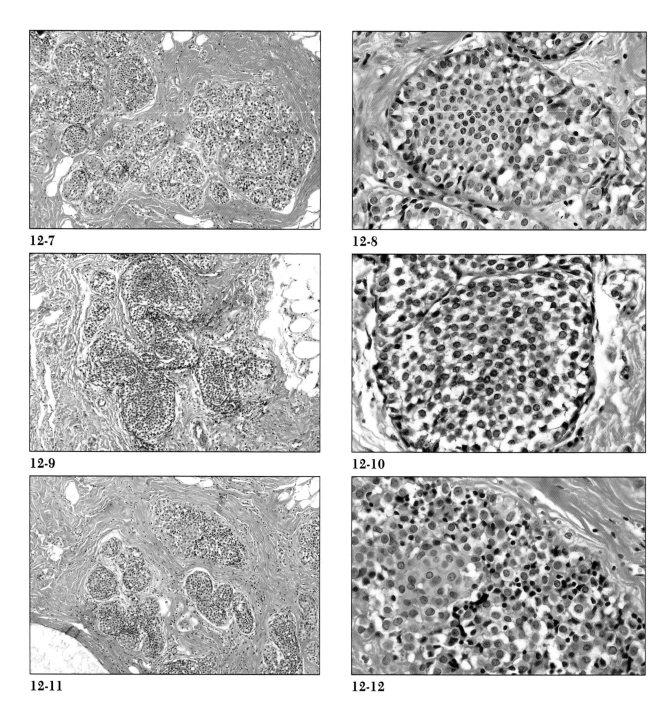

12-7

12-8

12-9

12-10

12-11

12-12

Figure 12-7. Lobular carcinoma in situ may consist of a mixture of large cells and small cells within the same or adjacent ductules.

Figure 12-9. This example of lobular carcinoma in situ has irregularly distributed cells without the "pavement stone" appearance often seen in this neoplasm.

Figure 12-11. Most of the ductules seen here contain typical lobular carcinoma in situ. The ductule at the upper right appears at this magnification to have a two-cell population.

Figure 12-8. A higher magnification of Figure 12-7 shows the small cell population with sharply demarcated cell borders. The larger cells, located peripherally, have fewer discrete cell borders.

Figure 12-10. A higher magnification of Figure 12-9 demonstrates that the monomorphic population of cells lacks well-defined cell borders.

Figure 12-12. A higher magnification of Figure 12-11 shows that the apparent two-cell population is due to focal degeneration with cell shrinkage and nuclear hyperchromasia. The intact cells retain the characteristic features of lobular carcinoma in situ.

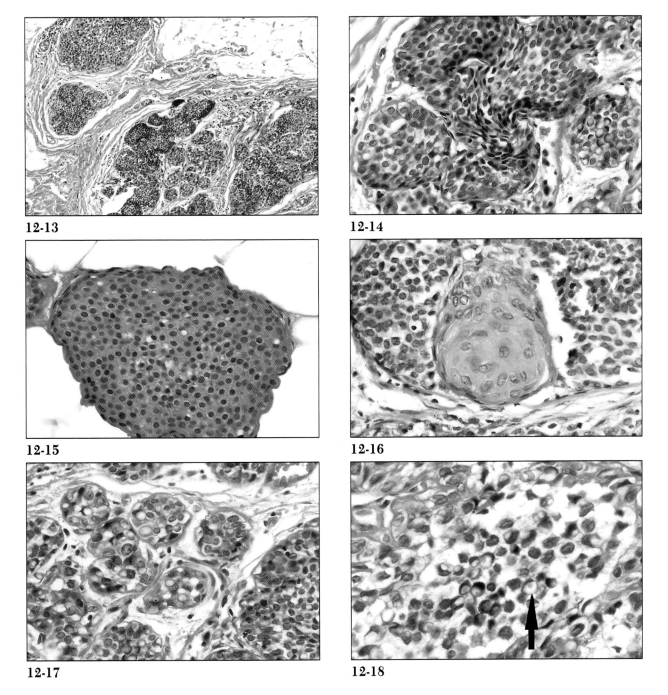

12-13

12-14

12-15

12-16

12-17

12-18

Figure 12-13. Lobular carcinoma in situ may have a variable appearance at low magnification due to differences in cell size and spacing.

Figure 12-15. Enlarged ductules of lobular carcinoma in situ are occasionally located in fat. Their sharp circumscription and lack of stromal response distinguish them from invasive carcinoma.

Figure 12-17. Lobular carcinoma in situ may consist of numerous cells with intracytoplasmic lumina of varying size.

Figure 12-14. A higher magnification of Figure 12-13 shows focal spindling of cells, presumably due to compression by adjacent proliferating cells. Neoplastic cells with intracytoplasmic lumina are especially prominent at right.

Figure 12-16. Rarely, nodules of squamous metaplasia may be seen in lobular carcinoma in situ. This is of no known prognostic importance and should not be interpreted as squamous cell carcinoma.

Figure 12-18. When the cells of lobular carcinoma in situ contain intracytoplasmic lumina with centrally placed, eosinophilic secretions (arrow), they are often referred to as "target cells."

LOBULAR CARCINOMA IN SITU

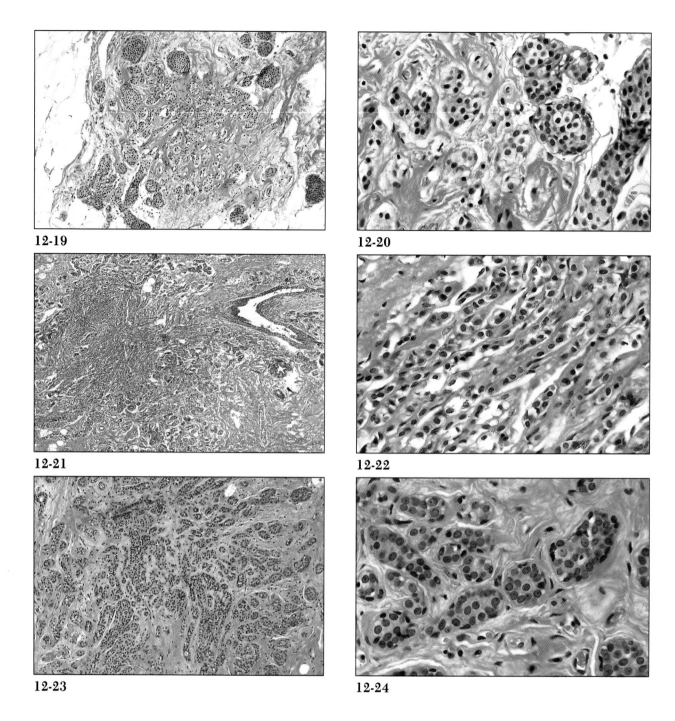

12-19

12-20

12-21

12-22

12-23

12-24

Figure 12-19. Lobular carcinoma in situ may involve foci of sclerosing adenosis. The larger ductules at the periphery are typical of sclerosing adenosis and are a helpful feature for distinguishing this lesion from invasive carcinoma.

Figure 12-21. This larger example of sclerosing adenosis with lobular carcinoma in situ maintains the overall pattern of the former lesion with better-formed ductules at the periphery.

Figure 12-23. This example of lobular carcinoma in situ in sclerosing adenosis has more widely separated ductules in a fibrotic stroma.

Figure 12-20. A higher magnification of the lesion in Figure 12-19 shows small, irregular aggregates and apparently single cells of lobular carcinoma. Emphasis on the overall architecture of sclerosing adenosis will avoid confusion of this in situ lesion with invasive carcinoma.

Figure 12-22. A higher magnification of the central portion of Figure 12-21 shows cords of lobular carcinoma in situ. This image, taken out of context, is indistinguishable from invasive carcinoma, except for the lack of a desmoplastic stromal response.

Figure 12-24. A higher magnification of Figure 12-23 shows that, although the ductules are not widely distended, they are populated by monomorphic neoplastic cells characteristic of lobular carcinoma.

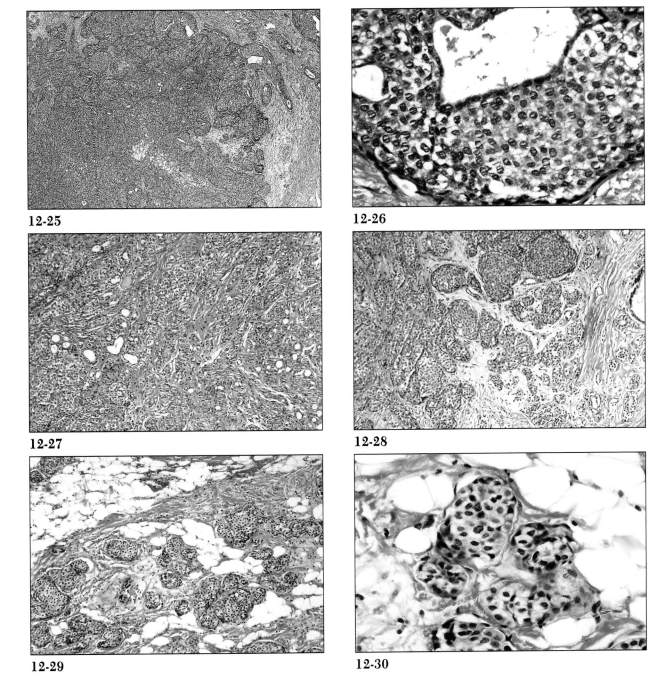

12-25

12-26

12-27

12-28

12-29

12-30

Figure 12-25. This example of lobular carcinoma in situ in sclerosing adenosis shows that the peripheral ductules may be greatly enlarged and abut one another with a negligible stromal component.

Figure 12-27. The central portion of the lesion seen in Figures 12-25 and 12-26 has ductules of sclerosing adenosis, some of which are involved by lobular carcinoma in situ. A fibrous stromal component separates the ductules.

Figure 12-29. The alveolar variant of infiltrating lobular carcinoma consists of sharply circumscribed, variably sized nests of cells. Some of the nests are in loose fibrous stroma and others are surrounded by fat.

Figure 12-26. A higher magnification of Figure 12-25 shows a greatly distended ductule with a residual lumen. The myoepithelial cell layer at lower right and the normal lining epithelium of the lumen are widely separated by a zone of neoplastic cells.

Figure 12-28. The periphery of the lesion seen in Figures 12-25 to 12-27 has small ductules partially or completely involved with lobular carcinoma in situ. These may represent adjacent lobules that are "recruited" as this complex proliferation enlarges.

Figure 12-30. A higher magnification of Figure 12-29 discloses nests of cells within the spectrum of lobular carcinoma.

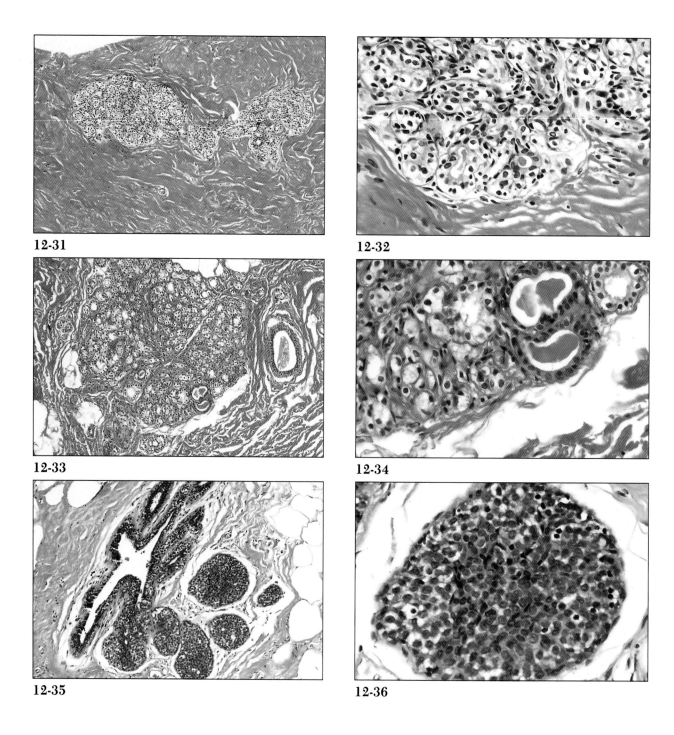

12-31

12-32

12-33

12-34

12-35

12-36

Figure 12-31. Lobules containing closely packed ductules involved by clear cell change may mimic lobular carcinoma in situ at low magnification.

Figure 12-33. This example of clear cell change involves one or more distorted lobules, possibly representing a small focus of sclerosing adenosis.

Figure 12-35. Epithelial hyperplasia of the usual type can greatly distend ductules.

Figure 12-32. A higher magnification of Figure 12-31 shows that the clear cell change involves myoepithelial cells in some ductules with preservation of the lumina (lower left). Other ductules lack a lumen, but are filled with polymorphous cells having angulated nuclei.

Figure 12-34. A higher magnification of Figure 12-33 shows two normal ductules containing secretory material and lacking clear cell change. Some ductules have clear cell change but retain a lumen. The distorted, small ductules at the left lack lumina, have clear cell change, and mimic lobular carcinoma.

Figure 12-36. A higher magnification of Figure 12-35 shows a polymorphic population of cells with angulated, overlapping nuclei.

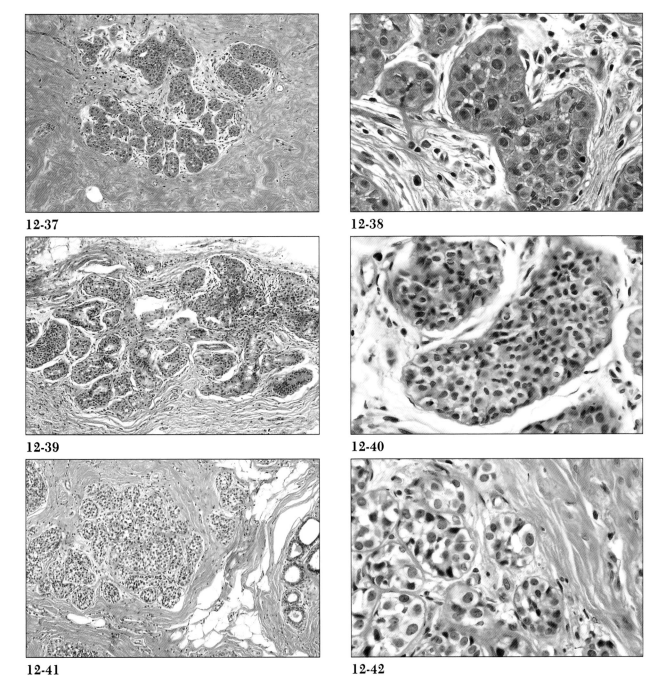

12-37

12-38

12-39

12-40

12-41

12-42

Figure 12-37. This example of epithelial hyperplasia involving ductules has larger cells with more prominent cytoplasm, as compared with Figure 12-35.

Figure 12-39. This lobular proliferation is characterized by slightly distended lobules that are partially populated by cells cytologically identical to lobular carcinoma in situ. Most of the lumina are maintained.

Figure 12-41. This lobular proliferation contains ductules located centrally that have obliterated lumina but no significant distention.

Figure 12-38. A higher magnification of Figure 12-37 shows cytologically variable cells with focally vacuolated, apocrine-like cytoplasm. This cytologic appearance does not fall within the spectrum of lobular carcinoma in situ or atypical lobular hyperplasia.

Figure 12-40. A higher magnification of Figure 12-39 shows ductules with obliterated lumina populated by cells having the powdery eosinophilic cytoplasm of lobular carcinoma in situ. Most cells, however, are polymorphic, varying in size and shape. Thus, this lesion is not atypical lobular hyperplasia as used by Page et al.

Figure 12-42. A higher magnification of Figure 12-41 shows that some cells in the ductule are within the spectrum of lobular carcinoma in situ. Other cells have angulated, dense nuclei and are not diagnostic of lobular neoplasia.

LOBULAR CARCINOMA IN SITU

162

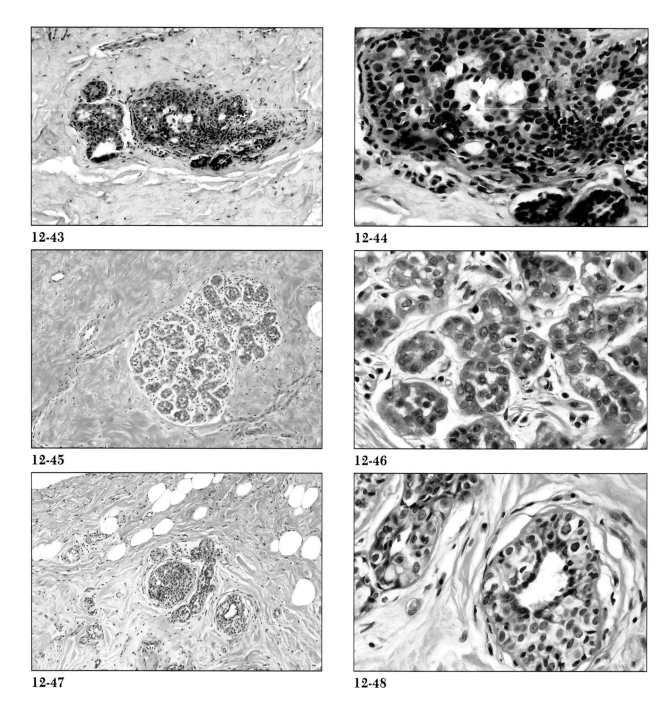

12-43

12-44

12-45

12-46

12-47

12-48

Figure 12-43. This lobular proliferation with minimal epithelial abnormalities consists of a markedly distorted aggregate of ductules and, possibly, the intralobular portion of the terminal duct.

Figure 12-45. Atypical lobular hyperplasia lacks ductular distension and has remnants of lumina in many ductules.

Figure 12-47. In this example of atypical lobular hyperplasia, two ductules are distended and one of these retains its lumen.

Figure 12-44. A higher magnification of Figure 12-43 shows individual cells with powdery cytoplasm (far left), as well as scattered cells with enlarged, hyperchromatic nuclei. The term *atypical lobular hyperplasia* can be applied to such a lesion, although the data of Page et al cannot be applied.

Figure 12-46. A higher magnification of Figure 12-45 confirms the presence of a monomorphic cell population.

Figure 12-48. A higher magnification of Figure 12-47 shows that the lumen in the distended ductule is rimmed by normal epithelium. Beneath this layer is a monomorphic population of neoplastic cells.

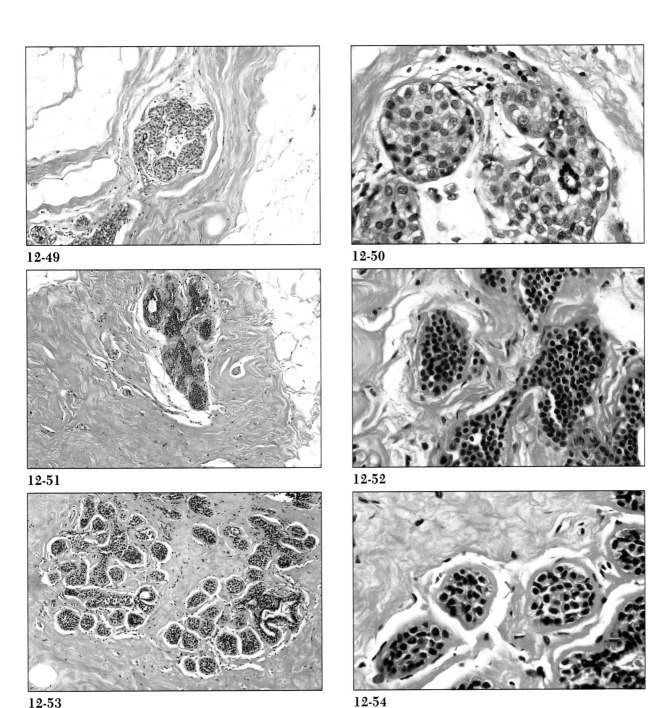

12-49

12-50

12-51

12-52

12-53

12-54

Figure 12-49. This lobule is interpreted as atypical lobular hyperplasia based on the presence of a monomorphic population of neoplastic cells within the spectrum of lobular carcinoma in situ, but occurring in the absence of ductular distension.

Figure 12-51. This small, seemingly atrophic lobule nonetheless has its ductules filled with a monomorphic population. We consider this to be a variant of atypical lobular hyperplasia that does not meet the criteria of Page et al for that diagnosis.

Figure 12-53. We interpret this as a variant of atypical lobular hyperplasia, although it lacks the criteria of Page et al for that diagnosis. Note the lack of ductular distension and the presence of well-formed lumina.

Figure 12-50. This higher magnification of Figure 12-49 shows a monomorphic population of cells except for a minute residual lumen lined by normal ductal epithelium. The difference in nuclear size between the neoplastic and normal cells can be easily appreciated.

Figure 12-52. A higher magnification of Figure 12-51 confirms the uniform appearance of the small neoplastic cells filling the ductules.

Figure 12-54. A higher magnification of Figure 12-53 shows that the monomorphic neoplastic cells are larger and have slightly more cytoplasm than in the case illustrated in Figure 12-46.

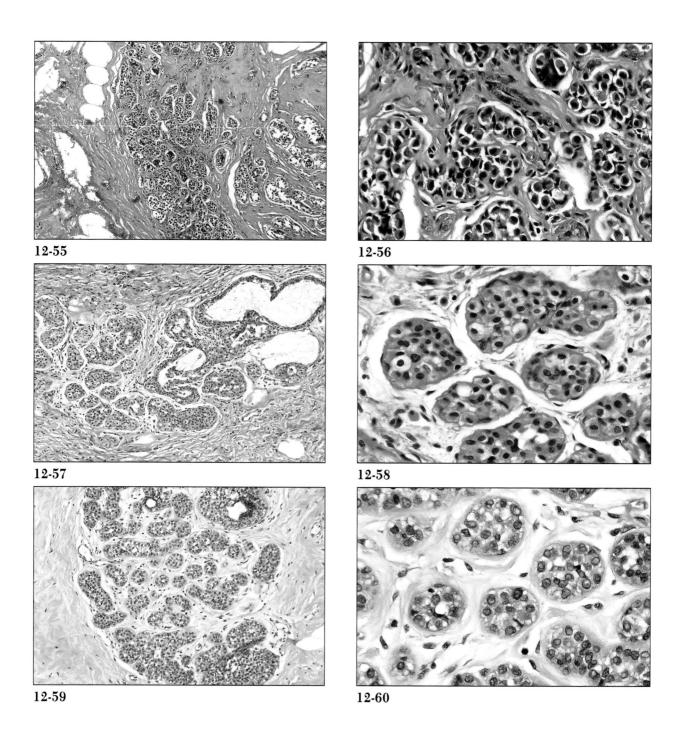

12-55

12-56

12-57

12-58

12-59

12-60

Figure 12-55. In this example of lobular hyperplasia, normal-sized ductules are filled with loosely cohesive cells.

Figure 12-57. This example of minimally atypical lobular proliferation consists of several normally sized or minimally distended ductules containing neoplastic cells within the spectrum of lobular carcinoma in situ (left). The ductules at right are filled with mucin, and do not resemble the solid proliferation of lobular carcinoma in situ.

Figure 12-59. This example of atypical lobular hyperplasia closely approaches the appearance of lobular carcinoma in situ. Because approximately one half of the ductules are not distended and others have residual lumina (top), we would not interpret this image as lobular carcinoma in situ.

Figure 12-56. A higher magnification of Figure 12-55 shows that the abnormal cells have a "plasmacytoid" appearance and are intermixed with smaller cells having angulated, elongated nuclei. This results in a Paget-like appearance in which isolated abnormal cells are retracted from the surrounding smaller cells.

Figure 12-58. A higher magnification of Figure 12-57 shows normal-sized ductules containing cells within the spectrum of lobular carcinoma in situ, and normal cells. There is not a sufficiently monomorphic population of cells nor sufficient ductular distention to qualify for atypical lobular hyperplasia as defined by Page et al.

Figure 12-60. A higher magnification of Figure 12-59 shows normal-sized ductules lacking lumina and containing neoplastic cells with vacuolated cytoplasm and the uniform, bubbly nuclei sometimes seen in lobular carcinoma in situ.

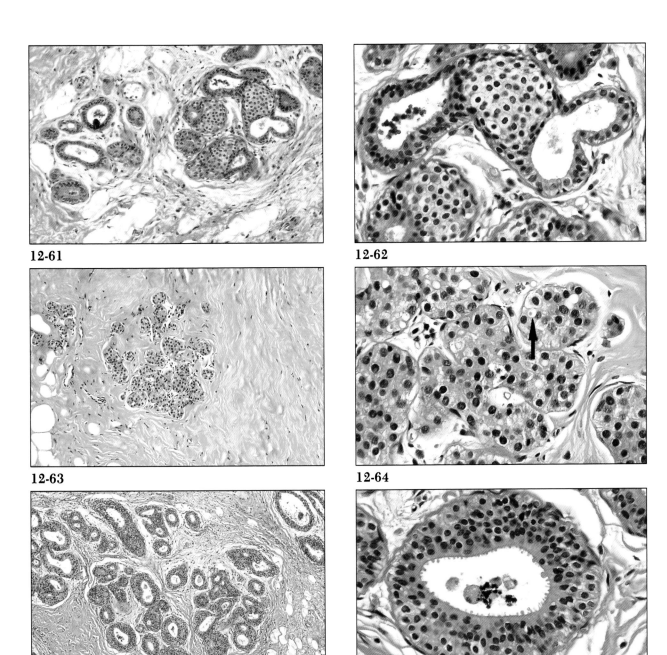

12-61

12-62

12-63

12-64

12-65

12-66

Figure 12-61. Another example of atypical lobular hyperplasia consists of ductules that are partially involved with cells typical of lobular neoplasia (right).

Figure 12-63. The normal-sized ductules in this example of atypical lobular hyperplasia are filled with a monomorphic population of cells within the spectrum of lobular carcinoma in situ.

Figure 12-65. These lobules have moderately distended ductules with preservation of lumina. We interpret this as an example of atypical lobular hyperplasia.

Figure 12-62. This higher magnification of Figure 12-61 shows normal epithelium partially lining the ductule and abutting a separate, monomorphic population with the cytologic features of lobular neoplasia.

Figure 12-64. A higher magnification of Figure 12-63 shows the monomorphic cell population of lobular carcinoma in situ, including characteristic "target cells" (arrow).

Figure 12-66. A higher magnification of Figure 12-65 shows a distended ductule lined by a thick mantle of monomorphic cells. The calcified debris in the lumen is a clue to the presence of either lobular or ductular neoplasia.

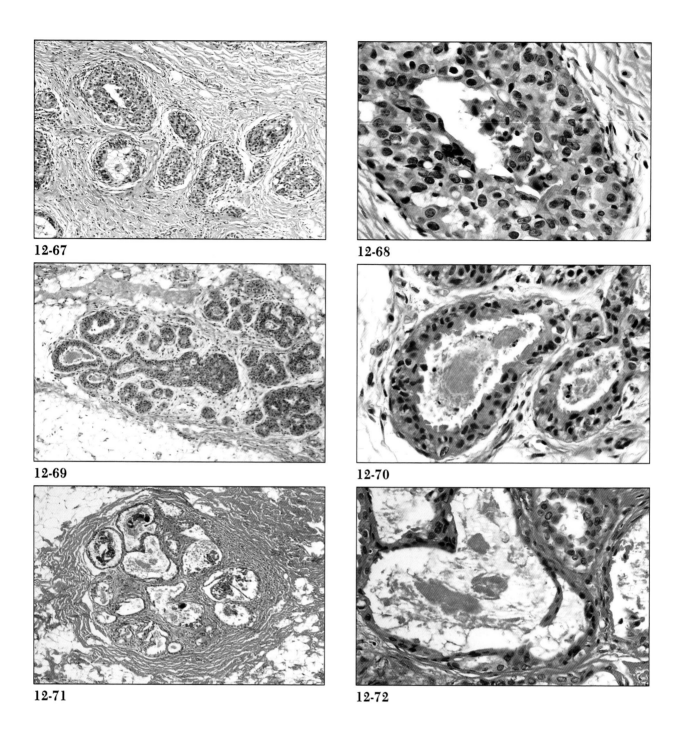

12-67

12-68

12-69

12-70

12-71

12-72

Figure 12-67. Some of the minimally distended ductules in this example of atypical lobular hyperplasia maintain their lumina.

Figure 12-69. A few moderately distended ductules (left) contain eosinophilic debris in their lumina. This patient had clear-cut comedocarcinoma in other microscopic fields.

Figure 12-71. This example of comedo-carcinoma involving a lobule has a minimal epithelial component and a large amount of calcified, necrotic luminal debris. Comedocarcinoma involving ducts was present elsewhere in this case.

Figure 12-68. A higher magnification of Figure 12-67 shows exfoliated, degenerating epithelial cells, raising the possibility of incipient comedonecrosis.

Figure 12-70. A higher magnification of Figure 12-69 shows comedonecrosis associated with cytologic atypia. Because of the clear-cut comedocarcinoma elsewhere in this case, we interpret this as involvement of ductules by comedocarcinoma (lobular "cancerization").

Figure 12-72. A higher magnification of Figure 12-71 shows small, focally flattened, but nonetheless atypical epithelial cells. Identical cells were present in the associated ductal comedocarcinoma.

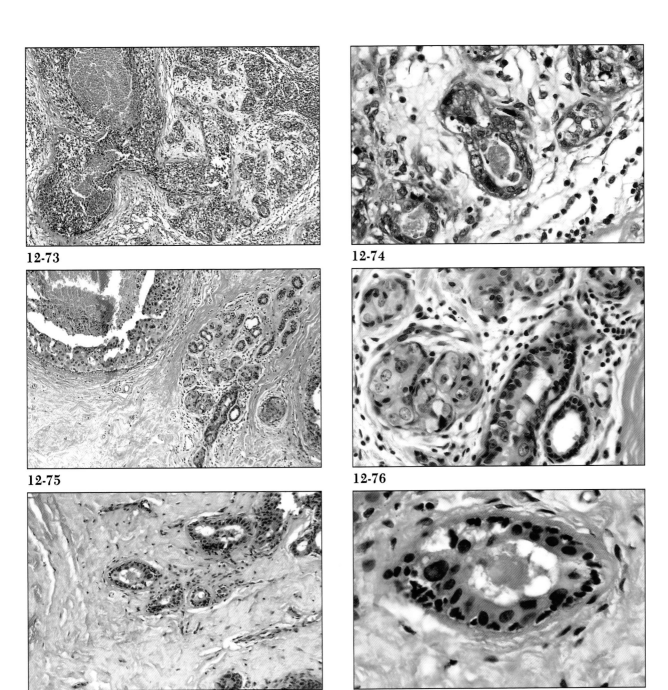

12-73

12-74

12-75

12-76

12-77

12-78

Figure 12-73. Comedocarcinoma involving a large duct (left) is in direct continuity with smaller ducts and ductules (right).

Figure 12-75. A large duct with comedocarcinoma is present at upper left. The adjacent lobule contains both normal ductules and ductules populated by atypical cells.

Figure 12-77. Another example of lobular involvement by comedocarcinoma has normal-sized ductules with subtle cytologic abnormalities at this magnification.

Figure 12-74. A higher magnification of the ductules from Figure 12-73 shows that some retain their lumina and have intraluminal necrotic debris. The ductules are lined by cytologically pleomorphic neoplastic cells identical to those of the comedocarcinoma.

Figure 12-76. A higher magnification of Figure 12-75 shows a normal ductule at the far right. The adjacent elongated ductule is partially populated by large, atypical cells. At the left are several closely apposed ductules almost completely filled with identical atypical cells.

Figure 12-78. A higher magnification of Figure 12-77 shows varying degrees of nuclear enlargement in the epithelial layer. At left is a markedly enlarged nucleus. The lumen contains dense eosinophilic material that may represent necrotic debris.

168

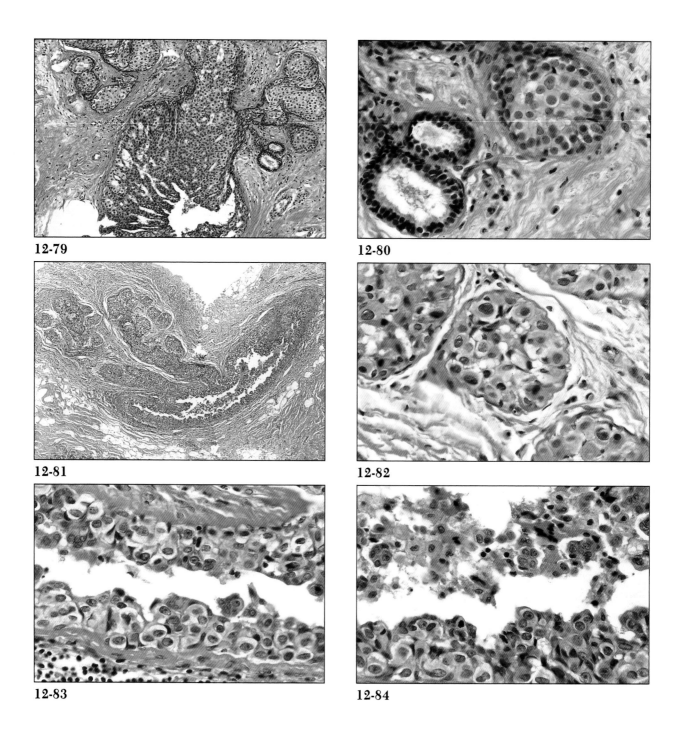

12-79

12-80

12-81

12-82

12-83

12-84

Figure 12-79. Both the ductules at the upper portion of the field and the larger duct located centrally are involved with the same population of uniform, neoplastic cells. The ductular component has all the features of lobular carcinoma in situ, and yet the cytologically identical intraductal cells have the micropapillary pattern of ductal carcinoma in situ.

Figure 12-81. Ductules at the upper left are diagnostic of lobular carcinoma in situ. Two terminal ducts, also involved with lobular carcinoma in situ, are in direct continuity with a subsegmental duct.

Figure 12-83. Another higher-power magnification of the subsegmental duct in Figure 12-81 shows a pagetoid-like change with flattened luminal epithelium visible focally.

Figure 12-80. A higher magnification of Figure 12-79 shows a distended ductule, diagnostic of lobular carcinoma in situ.

Figure 12-82. A higher magnification of Figure 12-81 shows ductules slightly distended by mildly pleomorphic cells diagnostic of lobular carcinoma in situ.

Figure 12-84. A higher magnification of Figure 12-81 shows exfoliated, degenerating epithelial cells suggestive of incipient comedonecrosis.

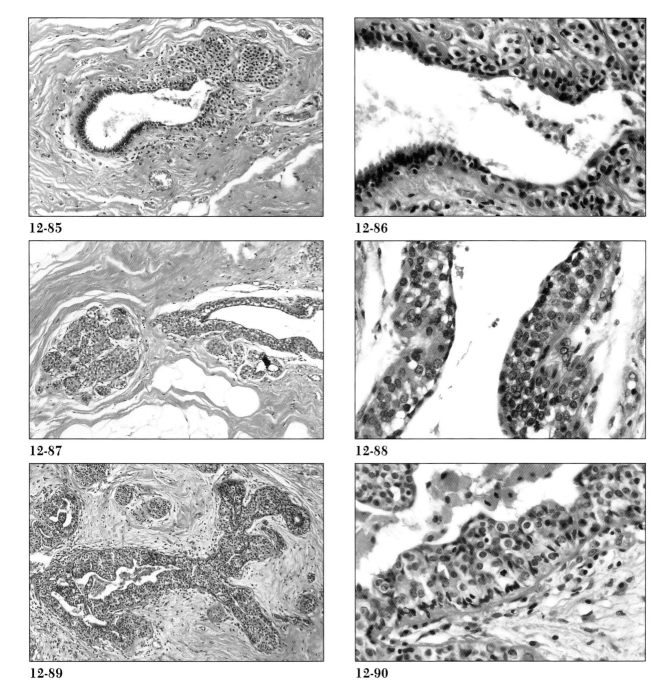

12-85

12-86

12-87

12-88

12-89

12-90

Figure 12-85. Lobular carcinoma in situ (right) is in direct continuity with cytologically identical cells involving the terminal duct. The distal portion of the terminal duct is lined by normal epithelium.

Figure 12-87. The combination of pagetoid change in the subsegmental duct (right) and atypical lobular hyperplasia (left) has clinical relevance, as discussed in the text.

Figure 12-89. When pagetoid change is several cells thick, it is often intermixed with nonneoplastic ductal cells.

Figure 12-86. A higher magnification of Figure 12-85 shows the involved terminal duct with residual, flattened luminal epithelium overlying nests and single neoplastic cells.

Figure 12-88. A higher magnification of Figure 12-87 shows a subsegmental duct with residual, flattened luminal epithelium and underlying pagetoid change.

Figure 12-90. A higher magnification of Figure 12-89 shows pagetoid cells with larger, predominantly round nuclei and distinct cell borders intermixed with nonneoplastic cells having smaller, predominantly angulated nuclei.

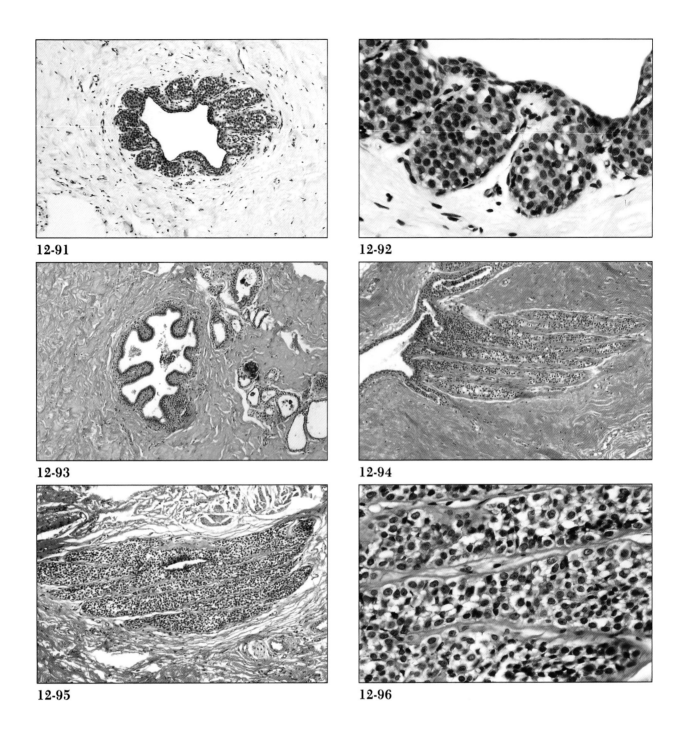

12-91

12-92

12-93

12-94

12-95

12-96

Figure 12-91. Ducts involved with pagetoid change often have a so-called cloverleaf pattern when sectioned transversely.

Figure 12-93. Normal subsegmental ducts may have an irregular, corrugated contour.

Figure 12-95. This tangential section of a markedly corrugated subsegmental duct demonstrates pagetoid change and has multiple, laminated cords of neoplastic cells.

Figure 12-92. A higher magnification of Figure 12-91 depicts sharply circumscribed aggregates of uniform, neoplastic cells.

Figure 12-94. A subsegmental duct of the same size and configuration as that seen in Figure 12-93 demonstrates pagetoid change. When cut tangentially, the corrugated portion appears as parallel cords of cells separated by fibrous tissue.

Figure 12-96. A higher magnification of Figure 12-95 verifies the presence of a cytologically distinctive population of neoplastic cells.

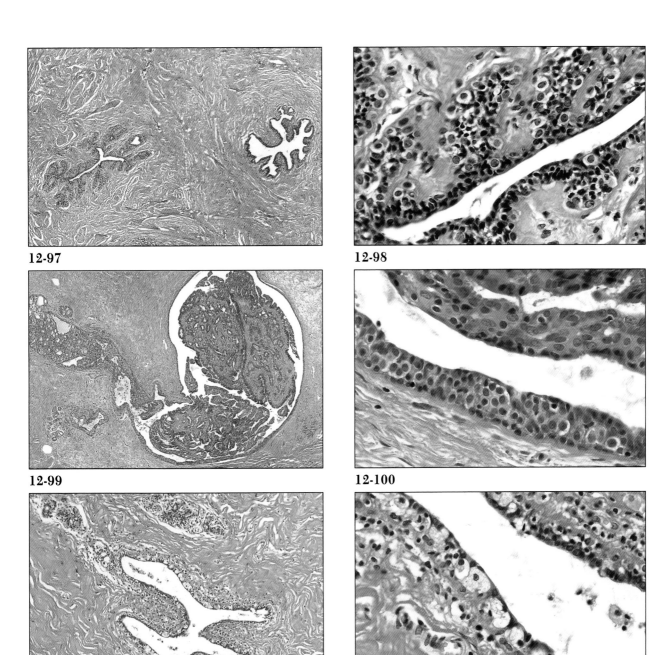

12-97

12-98

12-99

12-100

12-101

12-102

Figure 12-97. Pagetoid change may affect the lactiferous ducts (left). The lactiferous duct at the right is normal.

Figure 12-99. Pagetoid change can occur coincident with other ductal abnormalities. In this instance, pagetoid change (left) is associated with an intraductal papilloma.

Figure 12-101. Intraepithelial foamy histiocytes may resemble pagetoid change at low magnification.

Figure 12-98. A higher magnification of the duct on the left in Figure 12-97 shows neoplastic cells, predominantly growing singly, along outpouchings of the lactiferous duct. The flattened residual luminal epithelium is clearly visible.

Figure 12-100. A higher magnification of Figure 12-99 contrasts the predominantly round cells of pagetoid change (bottom) with the elongated cells of the papilloma (top).

Figure 12-102. A higher magnification of Figure 12-101 shows flattened luminal epithelium, identical to that seen in pagetoid change, overlying the histiocytes. The latter cells, unlike pagetoid cells, have small nuclei and abundant, foamy cytoplasm.

LOBULAR CARCINOMA IN SITU

KEY TO OPTIONAL SLIDE SET

Slide 1. Pseudoangiomatous stromal hyperplasia surrounds lobules. Clefts are prominent, imparting an infiltrating, vascular-like appearance (see Figure 4-3).

Slide 2. Stromal cells in the pseudoangiomatous clefts may show nuclear enlargement and, rarely, mitotic activity. Numerous delicate cytoplasmic strands bridge the bloodless clefts (see Figure 4-5).

Slide 3. The junction of lobular carcinoma in situ (right) with uninvolved fibroadenoma (left) is clearly seen. Partial involvement of this type is common (see Figure 5-17).

Slide 4. The lobular carcinoma in situ in this fibroadenoma demonstrates characteristic target cells (see Figure 5-18).

Slide 5. Juvenile fibroadenoma has more cellular stroma and more prominent epithelial hyperplasia than typical adult-type fibroadenoma. The low-power pattern, unlike adult-type fibroadenoma, resembles florid gynecomastia (see Figure 5-19).

Slide 6. At higher magnification, the epithelium of juvenile fibroadenoma forms looping bridges and vertical papillae. Exfoliated strips of epithelium are also present in the lumen (see Figure 5-22).

Slide 7. The proliferating ductal epithelium of nipple adenoma is contiguous with the squamous epithelium of the nipple surface (see Figure 6-1).

Slide 8. The epithelium of nipple adenoma displays the cytologic variation typical of usual-type hyperplasia (see Figure 6-4).

Slide 9. Necrosis may be seen occasionally in nipple adenoma. Note that the cells have the cytologic features of hyperplasia as seen in Slide 8 (see Figure 6-5).

Slide 10. The gross appearance of a radial scar is indistinguishable from that of a small infiltrating carcinoma. Note the chalky streaks in the center of the scar (see Figure 7-1).

Slide 11. The earliest change in a developing radial scar is, presumably, a proliferation of intralobular and interlobular myofibroblasts (see Figure 7-2).

Slide 12. A higher magnification of Slide 11 shows hypercellular fibrous tissue with more prominent collagen at the periphery of the cellular zone (see Figure 7-3).

Slide 13. Still higher magnification of Slide 11 shows plump fibroblastic nuclei with minimal atypia. Very little collagen is present in this region (see Figure 7-4).

Slide 14. Peripheral ductules in radial scar are often the largest in the lesion and may show intraductal hyperplasia (see Figure 7-11).

Slide 15. This example of usual-type hyperplasia in radial scar exhibits the nuclear variability characteristic of hyperplasia (see Figure 7-12).

Slide 16. The peripherally located ductules of sclerosing adenosis (left and top) tend to have larger diameters than those located centrally (lower right) (see Figure 7-13).

Slide 17. Ductules in sclerosing adenosis may form obvious lumina of varying sizes. Other duc-

174 tules appear as aggregates of cells with small or barely discernible lumina. Only the larger ductules have a clearly recognizable myoepithelial cell layer (see Figure 7-14).

Slide 18. Sclerosing adenosis may have extremely cellular areas with only rare lumina. Individual lobules are no longer apparent, and this illustration may represent several confluent lobules (see Figure 7-17).

Slide 19. A higher magnification of Slide 18 shows closely packed cells with mild nuclear pleomorphism. Although epithelial and myoepithelial components are probably present, they cannot be distinguished on H&E-stained sections (see Figure 7-18).

Slide 20. This adenosis tumor formed a mammographically detected lesion. The resected mass consists of closely approximated nodules of sclerosing adenosis (see Figure 7-25).

Slide 21. Another adenosis tumor shows haphazardly arranged but cytologically bland cells, some with spindled nuclei (see Figure 7-30).

Slide 22. Microglandular adenosis may have small ductule-like structures irregularly distributed around a large, subsegmental duct. Although many of the lumina are circular, others have more variable shapes (see Figure 7-37).

Slide 23. Ductule-like structures of microglandular adenosis haphazardly arranged in fat without any evidence of lobule formation (see Figure 7-38).

Slide 24. The epithelial lining of microglandular adenosis is most often composed of a single layer of uniform cells. Dense luminal secretions, as seen here, are commonly present (see Figure 7-39).

Slide 25. The tubular carcinoma shown here has ductule-like structures similar in size to those of microglandular adenosis. Many of the spaces, however, are ovoid or sharply angulated. Microglandular adenosis, in contrast, has ductule-like structures with smoother contours (see Figure 7-43).

Slide 26. The ductule-like structures of tubular carcinoma are frequently composed of cells with apocrine "snouts." Note the marked desmoplasia, in contrast with microglandular adenosis (see Figure 7-44).

Slide 27. An unfolding lobule contains a small intraductal papilloma (see Figure 8-1).

Slide 28. A higher magnification of the intraductal papilloma in Slide 27 discloses a delicate fibrovascular core. This feature distinguishes papillomas from epithelial hyperplasia of the usual type (see Figure 8-2).

Slide 29. This example of an atypical papilloma consists of a complex ductal papilloma containing several foci at the left of cytologically atypical cells (see Figure 8-5).

Slide 30. A higher magnification of the atypical papilloma in Slide 29 shows a monomorphic population of cells with well-defined cytoplasmic borders and powdery eosinophilic cytoplasm. This cell population is in marked contrast to the apocrine epithelium constituting the remainder of the papilloma (see Figure 8-6).

Slide 31. This large duct papilloma has well-defined, branching fibrovascular stalks. The irregular configuration of the papilloma leads to planes of section that appear to contain entrapped epithelium (see Figure 8-8).

Slide 32. Some papillomas contain dense epithelial cell nuclei with scant cytoplasm (top) (see Figure 8-10).

Slide 33. This infarcted papilloma has broad areas of fibrosis (right). Large areas of squamous metaplasia are also present (see Figure 8-23).

Slide 34. The squamous metaplasia in this infarcted papilloma contains cells that form keratin pearls and have active-appearing nuclei (see Figure 8-24).

Slide 35. This papilloma is partially replaced with ductal carcinoma in situ. Broad sheets of atypical cells lack a papillomatous architecture. The associated papillomatous component is seen at the right (see Figure 8-27).

Slide 36. A higher magnification of Slide 35 shows the juxtaposition of typical epithelium (right) and markedly atypical cells with enlarged vesicular nuclei (left) (see Figure 8-28).

Slide 37. The carcinomatous component seen in Slide 35 contains cells with atypical-appearing mitotic figures (see Figure 8-30).

Slide 38. This sharply circumscribed ductal adenoma has confluent nodules of sclerosing adenosis (bottom), papilloma (lower right), and a densely fibrotic, calcified area (see Figure 8-44).

Slide 39. Two ducts in continuity contain strikingly different images. The duct on the left is a papilloma, and the one on the right has all the characteristics of ductal adenoma (see Figure 8-47).

Slide 40. A higher magnification of Slide 39 shows the contiguity of the papilloma and ductal adenoma (see Figure 8-48).

Slide 41. An adenomyoepithelioma has a central proliferation of spindled myoepithelial cells and peripheral lumen-forming epithelial cells (see Figure 8-49).

Slide 42. The spectrum of myoepithelial cells in adenomyoepithelioma includes elongated forms with invisible cell borders, as well as loosely arranged cells with stellate cytoplasm (see Figure 8-52).

Slide 43. The cut surface of juvenile papillomatosis exhibits fibrous tissue, yellow and tan areas of epithelial proliferation, and cysts of varying sizes (see Figure 9-1).

Slide 44. Juvenile papillomatosis typically has elements of epithelial hyperplasia intermixed with cysts of varying size. Fibrous tissue surrounds the epithelial elements, as well as extending into surrounding fat (see Figure 9-2).

Slide 45. Moderate hyperplasia of usual type is an epithelial proliferation more than five cells thick. The epithelium can form bridges across the lumen or papillae (see Figure 10-27).

Slide 46. The thickened epithelium of moderate hyperplasia often forms papillae. The cells at the tips of papillae are frequently small with dense nuclei (see figure 10-28).

Slide 47. In florid hyperplasia, most of the lumen is replaced by epithelium, leaving irregular, often angulated spaces (see Figure 10-37).

Slide 48. A higher magnification of the florid hyperplasia in Slide 47 discloses overlapping nuclei and an irregular arrangement of cells around the residual luminal spaces (see Figure 10-38).

Slide 49. The epithelial proliferation of florid hyperplasia may fill most of the duct lumen (see Figure 10-39).

Slide 50. The papillae of florid hyperplasia lack a fibrovascular core, distinguishing them from papillomas (see Figure 10-40).

Slide 51. Irregular, lumen-like spaces in florid hyperplasia are lined by inconsistently oriented cells. Mitotic figures, as seen here, may be present in hyperplasia, but these always have a typical configuration (see Figure 10-42).

Slide 52. Florid hyperplasia may be an almost completely solid epithelial proliferation filling the duct. The lumen-like spaces that remain are concentrated at the periphery (see Figure 10-43).

Slide 53. The central portion of the florid hyperplasia seen in Slide 52 has irregularly distributed nuclei, resulting in small islands of cytoplasm without discernible cell borders (see Figure 10-44).

Slide 54. Another higher magnification of the florid hyperplasia in Slide 52 shows that the luminal epithelial cells are exfoliated as they degenerate. This should not be confused with comedocarcinoma (see Figure 10-45).

Slide 55. A higher magnification of Slide 52 shows that the cells in the deeper layers of florid hyperplasia have plump, "active" nuclei. The more superficial cells have small, contracted nuclei and less cytoplasm (see Figure 10-46).

Slide 56. This large duct with florid hyperplasia has numerous lumen-like spaces resembling cribriform ductal carcinoma in situ at low magnification (see Figure 10-51).

Slide 57. A higher magnification of Slide 56 illustrates the bland, variably sized nuclei of usual-type hyperplasia. The epithelial cells have no constant orientation with respect to the lumen-like spaces (see Figure 10-52).

Slide 58. Usual hyperplasia may form papillae and bridges that mimic micropapillary ductal carcinoma in situ (see Figure 10-55).

Slide 59. A higher magnification of the usual hyperplasia seen in Slide 58 shows that the "Roman bridges" of epithelium have ovoid, overlapping nuclei. The apocrine "snouts" seen here are of no value for distinguishing hyperplasia from carcinoma (see Figure 10-56).

Slide 60. This example of florid hyperplasia has numerous bridges of epithelium, resulting in irregularly shaped lumina that mimic a mixture of cribriform and micropapillary carcinoma (see Figure 10-57).

Slide 61. A higher magnification of Slide 60 again demonstrates the overlapping nuclei and lack of cell orientation around lumen-like spaces that typifies usual hyperplasia (see Figure 10-58).

Slide 62. This example of atypical hyperplasia has cells almost completely filling the duct lumen (see Figure 10-59).

Slide 63. Higher magnification of Slide 62 discloses a small opening near the bottom of the field, suggesting true lumen formation of the type seen in cribriform ductal carcinoma in situ. A few cells at lower right have sharply defined cell borders (see Figure 10-60).

Slide 64. At low magnification, this example of atypical hyperplasia has ducts that display the spectrum of appearances seen in usual florid hyperplasia, including irregular lumen-like spaces and almost completely filled ducts. The microcalcifications are of no diagnostic value (see Figure 10-61).

Slide 65. A higher magnification of Slide 64 shows that most cells have overlapping and ovoid nuclei characteristic of usual hyperplasia. Streaming of the hyperplastic cells is prominent at the lower right. However, two lumina are lined by cells with basally oriented nuclei. This orientation is identical to that of cribriform carcinoma. We interpret this field as an example of hyperplasia with atypia (see Figure 10-62).

Slide 66. Florid epithelial hyperplasia of the usual type may form bridges and papillae resembling micropapillary ductal carcinoma in situ at low magnification (see Figure 10-63).

Slide 67. A higher magnification of Slide 66 shows the ovoid, overlapping nuclei and cell "streaming" of hyperplasia (see Figure 10-64).

Slide 68. Another higher magnification of Slide 66 discloses papillae with irregularly arranged cells and cytologic variation typical of hyperplasia (see Figure 10-65).

Slide 69. A few cells from the florid hyperplasia seen in Slide 66 have increased amounts of powdery cytoplasm and enlarged nuclei. Cells of this type, when they form a monomorphic population, are characteristic of cribriform and micropapillary ductal carcinoma in situ. The biologic potential of these few cells is unknown (see Figure 10-66).

Slide 70. This intraductal proliferation has the appearance at low magnification of florid hyperplasia of the usual type (see Figure 10-67).

Slide 71. A higher magnification of Slide 70 shows irregular lumen-like spaces characteristic of hyperplasia. However, occasional large nuclei are seen in cells with sharply defined cell borders. We interpret this as atypical hyperplasia on the basis of these focal cytologic abnormalities. The criteria of Page et al for the diagnosis of atypical hyperplasia are not fully met. Therefore, the biologic potential for this lesion is unclear (see Figure 10-68).

Slide 72. A duct of hyperplasia with atypia contains a long, almost solid strand of monomorphic cells mixed with the characteristic cells of hyperplasia (see Figure 10-69).

Slide 73. A higher magnification of Slide 72 shows an island of predominantly monomorphic cells traversing the lumen. The monomorphic cells have powdery, eosinophilic cytoplasm and evenly spaced nuclei (see Figure 10-70).

Slide 74. This example of atypical hyperplasia has numerous cytologically abnormal cells (see Figure 10-71).

Slide 75. A higher magnification of Slide 74 shows cells with high nuclear-to-cytoplasmic ratios. The nuclei are irregular in shape and many are hyperchromatic. Other areas of the duct such as at lower left are lined by cells of usual-type hyperplasia (see Figure 10-72).

Slide 76. The cut surface of this breast specimen shows multiple light yellow nodules representing the necrosis-filled ducts of comedocarcinoma (see Figure 11-13).

Slide 77. The cells at the periphery of comedocarcinoma may have an irregular distribution, resulting in spaces that appear to be true lumina. The cells are moderately large and exhibit considerable cytologic uniformity (see Figure 11-14).

Slide 78. Ducts involved with comedocarcinoma may have only a thin layer of neoplastic cells, best seen at the right (see Figure 11-29).

Slide 79. A higher magnification of Slide 78 shows a thin layer of markedly pleomorphic cells. There is full-thickness necrosis of the epithelium at the right. A myoepithelial cell layer is present for most of the ductal circumference (see Figure 11-30).

Slide 80. Closely approximated ducts and smaller ductules contain micropapillary ductal carcinoma in situ (see Figure 11-38).

Slide 81. The bridges of micropapillary ductal carcinoma in situ are composed of a monomorphic population of cells. There is no "streaming" of the epithelial cells within the bridge (see Figure 11-40).

Slide 82. This resection specimen containing micropapillary ductal carcinoma in situ has widely dilated, tan ducts filled with neoplastic epithelium (see Figure 11-45).

Slide 83. The closely apposed ducts of micropapillary ductal carcinoma in situ have lumina almost filled with neoplastic cells, accounting for the gross appearance in Slide 82 (see Figure 11-46).

Slide 84. A higher magnification of Slide 83 shows complex epithelial proliferations. For the most part, the nuclei are evenly spaced and the cells are oriented along the lumina without "streaming" (see Figure 11-47).

Slide 85. These ducts contain micropapillary ductal carcinoma in situ with extensive, transluminal bridges (see Figure 11-67).

Slide 86. A higher magnification of Slide 85 shows larger neoplastic cells peripherally and smaller cells centrally. This results in a bimorphic appearance, although intermediate-sized cells are also present. These features suggest that a monomorphic population is present, although there is atrophy of the centrally located cells (see Figure 11-68).

Slide 87. The ducts of cribriform ductal carcinoma in situ contain neoplastic cells that make well-formed, true lumina (see Figure 11-79).

Slide 88. A higher magnification of Slide 87 shows an essentially monomorphic population of neoplastic epithelial cells. The presence of rare larger cells does not detract from this interpretation. The neoplastic cells are radially oriented around spaces, forming true glandular lumina (see Figure 11-80).

Slide 89. This markedly distended duct with carcinoma in situ resembles a ductal adenoma at low magnification. Many lumina are discernible. Ducts of this size may have fibrovascular septa, as seen here, separating aggregates of cribriform carcinoma (see Figure 11-85).

Slide 90. When ductal carcinoma in situ contains many lumina of varying shapes, and sizes separated by only a few neoplastic cells, the distinction between cribriform and micropapillary variants becomes arbitrary (see Figure 11-91).

Slide 91. A higher magnification of Slide 90 demonstrates that the periluminal cells are less well oriented than in typical cribriform ductal carcinoma in situ (see Figure 11-92).

Slide 92. In contrast to the previous examples, solid ductal carcinoma in situ need not completely fill the affected duct (see Figure 11-107).

Slide 93. A higher magnification of Slide 92 shows a monomorphic, although moderately pleomorphic, population of cells. Contrast the neoplastic cells with the normal epithelium lining the duct at the right (see Figure 11-108).

Slide 94. Papillary ductal carcinoma in situ is distinguished from other forms of ductal carcinoma in situ by the presence of fibrovascular stalks. In this example from deep within the breast, multiple ducts are involved (see Figure 11-121).

Slide 95. A higher magnification of Slide 94 shows pseudostratified layers of monomorphic cells with elongated nuclei. The complex papillae may appear as bridges or apparently dissociated cell nests in certain planes of section (see Figure 11-122).

Slide 96. Ductal carcinoma in situ has an angular protrusion of epithelium at the right. The possibility of microinvasion is suggested (see Figure 11-141).

Slide 97. A higher magnification of Slide 96 shows that, despite the discohesive nature of the cells and their denser nuclei, the epithelial-stromal junction is sharp. This is not interpreted as microinvasion (see Figure 11-142).

Slide 98. Intracystic carcinoma has a granular cyst lining in the central portion of the figure that contrasts with the predominantly smooth wall seen elsewhere (see Figure 11-145).

Slide 99. The granularity of the cyst wall is caused by multiple foci of micropapillary carcinoma (see Figure 11-147).

Slide 100. Ductal carcinoma in situ must be distinguished from mucocele-like lesion of the breast, seen here. Some of the mucin-filled ducts may retain an intact, flattened epithelial lining (left). Other ducts have their epithelial lining replaced by histiocytes (right) (see Figure 11-159).

Slide 101. A higher magnification of Slide 100 shows that the lining epithelium of the cyst wall has been replaced by mononucleated and multinucleated histiocytes containing mucin. The free-floating cells are muciphages and not epithelial cells (see Figure 11-160).

Slide 102. This example of lobular carcinoma in situ involves minimally dilated ductules (see Figure 12-1).

Slide 103. A higher magnification of Slide 102 discloses that the ductules are filled with a single population of small cells exhibiting only slight cytologic variation (see Figure 12-2).

Slide 104. This more florid example of lobular carcinoma in situ involves ductules that vary from minimally to widely dilated (see Figure 12-3).

Slide 105. A higher magnification of Slide 104 shows a slightly pleomorphic population of larger neoplastic cells, as compared with Slide 103. The mitotic figure at upper left is a rare finding in lobular carcinoma in situ. The four neoplastic cells at lower left are not microinvasive carcinoma (see Figure 12-4).

Slide 106. This example of lobular carcinoma in situ consists of cells with scant cytoplasm and unrecognizable cell borders (see Figure 12-5).

Slide 107. This lobular carcinoma in situ consists of cells with abundant, powdery cytoplasm and distinct cell borders. A few myoepithelial cells with spindled nuclei are compressed at the periphery of the ductule (see Figure 12-6).

Slide 108. Lobular carcinoma in situ may consist of numerous cells with intracytoplasmic lumina of varying size (see Figure 12-17).

Slide 109. When the cells of lobular carcinoma in situ contain intracytoplasmic lumina with centrally placed, eosinophilic secretions (arrow), they are often referred to as "target cells" (see Figure 12-18).

Slide 110. Lobular carcinoma in situ may involve foci of sclerosing adenosis. The overall pattern of sclerosing adenosis is maintained with well-formed ductules at the periphery (see Figure 12-21).

Slide 111. A higher magnification of the central portion of Slide 110 shows cords of lobular carcinoma in situ. This image, taken out of context, is indistinguishable from invasive carcinoma, except for the lack of a desmoplastic stromal response (see Figure 12-22).

Slide 112. This example of epithelial hyperplasia involving ductules has large cells with more prominent cytoplasm (see Figure 12-37).

Slide 113. A higher magnification of the epithelial hyperplasia involving ductules seen in Slide 112 shows cytologically variable cells with focally vacuolated, apocrine-like cytoplasm. This cytologic appearance does not fall within the spectrum of lobular carcinoma in situ or atypical lobular hyperplasia (see Figure 12-38).

Slide 114. This example of atypical lobular hyperplasia is characterized by slightly distended lobules that are partially populated by cells cytologically identical to lobular carcinoma in situ. Most of the lumina are maintained (see Figure 12-39).

Slide 115. A higher magnification of Slide 114 shows ductules with obliterated lumina populated by cells having the powdery eosinophilic cytoplasm of lobular carcinoma in situ. Most of the cells, however, are polymorphic, with considerable variation in size and shape. Therefore, this lesion falls short of the diagnosis of atypical lobular hyperplasia as used by Page et al (see Figure 12-40).

Slide 116. This example of atypical lobular hyperplasia contains ductules located centrally that have obliterated lumina but no significant distention (see Figure 12-41).

Slide 117. A higher magnification of Slide 116 shows that some of the cells filling the ductule are within the spectrum of lobular carcinoma in situ. Other cells, however, have angulated, dense nuclei and are not diagnostic of lobular neoplasia (see Figure 12-42).

Slide 118. Comedocarcinoma involving a large duct (left) is in direct continuity with smaller ducts and ductules (right) (see Figure 12-73).

Slide 119. A higher magnification from Slide 118 of the ductules involved by comedocarcinoma shows that some retain their lumina and have intraluminal necrotic debris. The ductules are lined by cytologically pleomorphic neoplastic cells identical to those of the comedocarcinoma (see Figure 12-74).

Slide 120. A large duct with comedocarcinoma is present at upper left. The adjacent lobule contains both normal ductules and ductules populated by atypical cells (see Figure 12-75).

Slide 121. A higher magnification of Slide 120 shows a normal ductule at the far right. The adjacent elongated ductule is partially populated by large, atypical cells. At the left are several closely apposed ductules almost completely filled with identical atypical cells (see Figure 12-76).

Slide 122. Lobular carcinoma in situ (right) is in direct continuity with cytologically identical cells involving the terminal duct. The distal portion of the terminal duct is lined by normal epithelium (see Figure 12-85).

Slide 123. A higher magnification of the lobular carcinoma in situ seen in Slide 122 shows the involved terminal duct with residual, flattened luminal epithelium overlying nests and single neoplastic cells (see Figure 12-86).

Slide 124. When pagetoid change is several cells thick, it is often intermixed with nonneoplastic ductal cells (see Figure 12-89).

Slide 125. A higher magnification of Slide 124 shows pagetoid cells with larger, predominantly round nuclei and distinct cell borders intermixed with nonneoplastic cells having smaller, predominantly angulated nuclei (see Figure 12-90).

Slide 126. Ducts involved with pagetoid change often have a so-called cloverleaf pattern when sectioned transversely (see Figure 12-91).

Slide 127. A higher magnification of the pagetoid change seen in Slide 126 depicts sharply circumscribed aggregates of uniform, neoplastic cells (see Figure 12-92).

INDEX

Numbers in **boldface** refer to pages on which illustrations appear.